Fast Facts

CW00722921

Fast Facts
Chronic and
Cancer Pain

Second edition

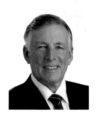

Michael J Cousins AM MD DSc FFPMANZCA FRCA
FANZCA FAChPM(RACP) FAICD
Professor and Head, Pain Management Research Institute
Royal North Shore Hospital
University of Sydney
New South Wales, Australia

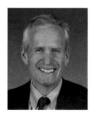

Rollin M Gallagher MD MPH DABPM FAAPM FAPA
Clinical Professor of Psychiatry and Anesthesiology and
Director for Pain Policy Research and Primary Care
Penn Pain Medicine, University of Pennsylvania
Deputy National Program Director for Pain Management
Veterans Health Administration and Pain Service
Philadelphia VA Medical Center
Philadelphia, USA

Declaration of Independence
This book is as balanced and as practical as we can make it.
Ideas for improvement are always welcome: feedback@fastfacts.com

HEALTH PRESS

Fast Facts: Chronic and Cancer Pain
First published 2007; reprinted with revisions 2008
Second edition March 2011

Text © 2011 Michael J Cousins, Rollin M Gallagher
© 2011 in this edition Health Press Limited
Health Press Limited, Elizabeth House, Queen Street, Abingdon,
Oxford OX14 3LN, UK
Tel: +44 (0)1235 523233
Fax: +44 (0)1235 523238

Book orders can be placed by telephone or via the website.
For regional distributors or to order via the website, please go to:
www.fastfacts.com
For telephone orders, please call +44 (0)1752 202301 (UK, Europe and Asia–
Pacific), 1 800 247 6553 (USA, toll free) or +1 419 281 1802 (Americas).

Fast Facts is a trademark of Health Press Limited.

A CIP record for this title is available from the British Library.

ISBN 978-1-905832-85-9

Cousins MJ (Michael)
Fast Facts: Chronic and Cancer Pain/
Michael J Cousins, Rollin M Gallagher

Medical illustrations by Annamaria Dutto, Withernsea, UK.
Typesetting and page layout by Zed, Oxford, UK.
Printed in China with Xpedient Print Services.

Introduction

All clinicians, regardless of specialty, will see patients with pain that has persisted for more than 6 months. It is now clear that persistent pain is a disease entity with a broad range of physical, psychological and environmental maladaptions involving the peripheral and central nervous systems. Thus, assessment and treatment of chronic pain is most effectively carried out in a biopsychosocial framework, drawing on a range of health professionals with knowledge and skills to enable them to address each of the three domains. Such professionals need to work in an interdisciplinary manner – communicating their findings face to face to permit them to weigh up the relative contributions of each domain. Chronic pain is not tabulated as a separate diagnosis in the World Health Organization's comprehensive estimates of global health burdens associated with highly prevalent conditions. Yet it is through chronic pain that many of the greatest global health burdens – cancer, HIV/AIDS, diabetes, arthritis, alcoholism and trauma (including war) – exact their long-term human, social and economic toll. Mental health problems such as anxiety and depression also place sufferers at increased risk of developing chronic pain, while those with chronic pain are prone to develop new anxiety or depression.

Chronic pain has not been a health priority until very recently. However, in Australia, USA, UK and mainland Europe major studies have shown that, on average, one person in five suffers chronic pain, with 30% severely disabled by it. The associated large financial costs, often borne over a lifetime, make chronic pain the third most costly health problem. The severe and unnecessary suffering is being brought to governmental attention by major initiatives ('Summits') of consumers and health professionals. Access to pain management as a Human Right is gaining considerable momentum. New hope for chronic pain sufferers has come from important advances in the understanding of mechanisms of chronic pain leading to new treatments aimed at a wide range of novel targets.

Fast Facts: Chronic and Cancer Pain describes a variety of chronic pain syndromes, discusses their pathogenesis and treatment(s) and provides the evidence for treatment effectiveness. This highly readable handbook provides a concise introduction to the complex and extensive field of chronic pain – it does not aim to be comprehensive. It seeks to distill a great deal of pain-related evidence, much of which cannot be synthesized mathematically because of the poor quality of many pain trials and the wide range of outcomes assessed across trials. Therefore, we have not attempted to tabulate the specific evidence supporting each therapeutic intervention, but have adopted the current practice in clinical decision-making of using clinical trial literature as 'tools not rules' and to practice 'evidence-guided' rather than 'evidence-based' medicine.

Fast Facts: Chronic and Cancer Pain is aimed primarily at the wide range of busy health professionals who are well aware that they have experienced little or no education and training to help them manage patients with chronic pain. Such practitioners include: those working at the primary care level (medical general practitioners, physical therapists, clinical psychologists, nurses, occupational therapists, pharmacists and many others), and also medical specialists across many specialties, apart from the new specialty of pain medicine.

The extraordinary situation where such a book is necessary has come about as a result of major ongoing deficiencies in education and training about pain, at an undergraduate level and in the majority of postgraduate healthcare training programs. Thus, healthcare undergraduates will find this book helpful as their first exposure to chronic pain. Also, pain medicine trainees/fellows may make use of the book at the beginning of their training to gain an overview of the area.

Acknowledgments

As clinicians and teachers we recognize the multidisciplinary and interdisciplinary nature of chronic pain and those who treat it. This book is dedicated to: our families, in grateful acknowledgment of their support during our often long hours; our colleagues, who have shared and thereby lightened our own professional burdens; and our patients and their families, who have sought to reclaim lives taken from them by chronic pain. We also thank Dan Carr and Soledad Cepeda who 'set the scene' in the first edition of this book.

Defining pain

There are many ways to classify pain; for example, by duration, etiology or intensity (Table 1.1). As understanding of the cellular mechanisms of pain has increased, proposals have been advanced to classify pain according to the predominant pathophysiological mechanism thought to be involved.

Present-day pain research was heralded by the publication of Melzack and Wall's 'gate control theory' in 1965, which provided a model for the modulation of incoming nociceptive information by the

TABLE 1.1

Possible ways of classifying pain

By duration	By probable mechanism
• Acute	• Tissue damage
• Subacute	• Inflammation
• Chronic	• Central sensitization of nociceptors
	• Nerve-damage-triggered neuroplasticity changes
By etiology	• Glia-derived neural sensitization
• Cancerous	• Loss of inhibition
• Ischemic	• Brain neuroplasticity changes
• Postoperative	• 'Cross-talk' between sympathetic and sensory neurons
By intensity	**By type of injured tissue**
• Mild	• Nociceptive
• Moderate	• Neuropathic
• Severe	• Visceral
	• Somatic

central nervous system (CNS). After publication of that model, researchers never again viewed the peripheral nervous system (PNS) or CNS as collections of cables passively transmitting nociceptive information.

The nervous system is dynamic; it is plastic, in that its structure and function are shaped and reshaped by activity within it, and at each level it continually amplifies or inhibits the signals that the brain ultimately interprets as pain. This plasticity is fundamental to the understanding of both the perpetuation of pain in some pain syndromes and the mechanisms of action of pain treatment modalities. There is large variability in the neuroplasticity response among individuals, and this accounts for the large variability in pain response (see below). For example, after surgery or trauma some patients suffer much higher than average acute pain levels. Importantly, these are the people who are at high risk of progression to persistent (chronic) pain.

Mechanisms of pain

It is universally recognized that factors in three domains contribute to the human experience of chronic pain: biological (nociceptive and neuropathic); psychological; and social (environmental). In fact, all three domains almost certainly exert their influence at various levels of the nervous system, with much overlap.

Biological. A stimulus of intensity sufficient to threaten tissue damage activates nociceptors, which are specialized nerve endings. A major advance has been the discovery of the transduction process of noxious temperature (heat and cold) and chemical stimuli, to generate electrical energy that conducts along the axon to the spinal cord. The transduction process for the remaining category of noxious stimuli associated with pressure will likely soon be elucidated. Existing knowledge of temperature and chemical mechanisms includes the key role of transient receptor potential vanilloid (TRPV), acid-sensing ion channel (ASIC) and P_2X receptor sites, which have become exciting new targets to block nociception at a peripheral level (Figure 1.1). The cell bodies of these nociceptors (first-order neurons) are located outside the spinal cord in the dorsal root ganglia and extend their

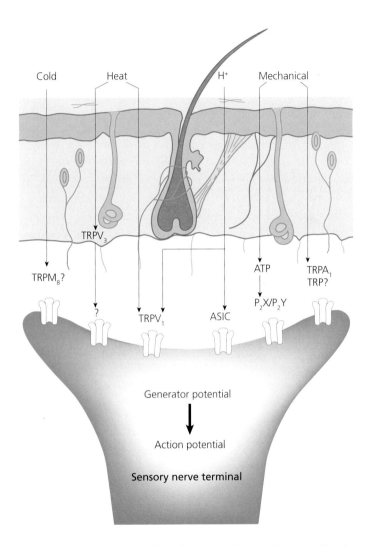

Figure 1.1 Peripheral transduction of pain. Noxious mechanical stimuli release ATP, which may act on one or more purine receptors (P_2X and P_2Y). A second mechanism may involve transient receptor potential (TRP) A_1 or other TRP receptors. Noxious chemical stimuli such as acidity (H^+) act via acid-sensing ion channels (ASICs) or TRP vanilloid $(TRPV)_1$ receptors. Noxious heat acts via $TRPV_1$ and $TRPV_2$, possibly via $TRPV_3$ receptors. Noxious cold acts via TRP melastatin $(TRPM)_8$ receptors. Based on Marchand et al. *Nat Rev Neurosci* 2005;6:521–32.

dendritic processes to the periphery. Activation of nociceptors triggers a volley of incoming impulses that travel to the spinal cord along both myelinated (Aδ) and unmyelinated (C) nerve fibers. These fibers enter the spinal cord almost exclusively through the dorsal root, and synapse in the dorsal horn of the spinal cord, where they project to higher levels such as the thalamus, hypothalamus, reticular system and cortex of the brain (Figure 1.2).

Roughly speaking, the higher-level sites bring about the aversive emotional feelings (thalamus and limbic system), alterations in sleep pattern (reticular system and hypothalamus) and stress responses (hypothalamus) that pain may evoke.

The PNS and CNS do not passively transduce stimuli and convey sensory information. Instead, noxious stimuli trigger biological processes that then amplify or inhibit the noxious signal.

Potentiation. After tissue or nerve damage, peripheral nociceptors become sensitized to noxious stimuli owing to the formation and accumulation of algogenic and inflammatory mediators in the periphery, such as prostanoids, interleukins, bradykinin and histamine. Peripheral sensitization and heightened afferent activity in pain fibers elicit functional, chemical and anatomic reorganization in spinal cord neurons. These changes lead to long-term central potentiation, a form of pain memory characterized by progressively enhanced and prolonged spinal neuronal responses to afferent impulses.

This spatially and temporally exaggerated processing of persistent nociceptive information translates clinically into increased experience of pain – not only response to noxious stimulation in the injured tissue (primary hyperalgesia), but also response in the surrounding uninjured tissue (secondary hyperalgesia), with repetitive stimulation producing progressively greater neuronal responses.

Central potentiation is due to the release by spinal afferent nociceptive neurons of excitatory mediators such as substance P and glutamate that bind to neurokinin 1 (NK1) and N-methyl D-aspartate (NMDA) receptors, respectively, in the dorsal horn. Concurrent activation of these receptors allows a massive influx of calcium into second-order neurons, the cell bodies of which lie within the dorsal

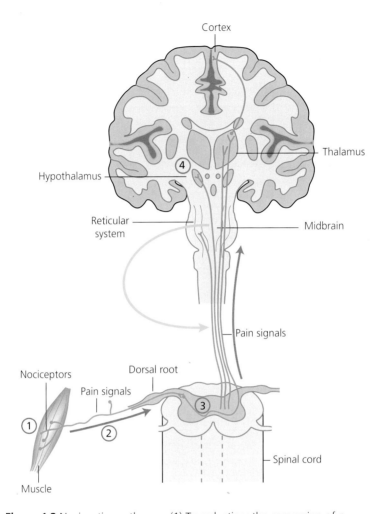

Figure 1.2 Nociceptive pathways. (1) Transduction: the conversion of a noxious stimulus into electrical energy by a peripheral nociceptor. (2) Transmission: propagation of the signal through the peripheral nervous system via first-order neurons. (3) Modulation: adjustment of pain intensity at the point where first-order neurons synapse with second-order neurons in the dorsal horn of the spinal cord. (4) Perception: the cerebral cortical response to nociceptive signals projected to the brain by third-order neurons. Stimulation of the descending pathway from the brain (green arrow) sends inhibitory responses back to the periphery – the brain can order the release of chemicals with an analgesic effect that may reduce or even abolish some forms of pain.

horn of the spinal cord. Consequently, calcium-dependent intracellular enzymes such as protein kinase C (PKC) are activated, catalyzing the production of nitric oxide (NO) and prostaglandins. These protein kinases also activate other proteins such as ion channels and enzymes (Figure 1.3).

Inhibition. Pain also triggers processes that dampen the perception of nociceptive stimuli. Nociceptive afferent traffic ascends to the midbrain and brainstem, where it activates descending pathways that inhibit spinal pain transmission (see Figure 1.2). These descending inhibitory systems are stimulated by endogenous opioids, as well as monoamines such as norepinephrine (noradrenaline) and serotonin. They inhibit spinal nociceptive transmission through the local release of inhibitory transmitters such as γ-aminobutyric acid (GABA), glycine, adenosine and endogenous opioids at the spinal level. Analgesics such as opioids and tricyclic antidepressants, in addition to their other mechanisms of action, activate these inhibitory systems. Furthermore, pain elicits a stress hormone response that includes the systemic secretion of endogenous opioids from the anterior pituitary and the adrenal medulla.

Interpretation

Pain is more than the nociceptive cascade described above. Pain is 'an unpleasant sensory and emotional experience associated with actual or potential tissue damage, or described in terms of such damage' (International Association for the Study of Pain [IASP]). Because it is an experience, pain itself cannot be measured directly. Pain, like consciousness itself, is constructed by complex brain processes that are strongly affected by a person's attitudes, beliefs, personality and interpretation of the significance of nociceptive stimuli. Central to the understanding of clinical pain is the concept that pain may be present without an obvious source or cause.

Mechanisms of neuropathic pain

Definition. Neuropathic pain is initiated or caused by a primary lesion of the PNS or CNS. Patients often complain not only of spontaneous

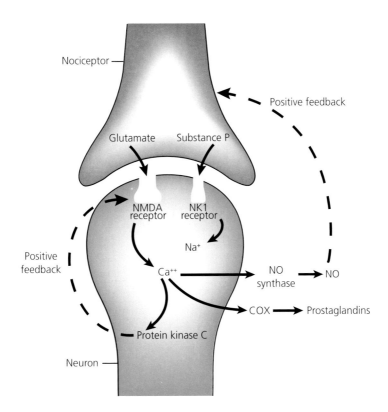

Figure 1.3 Central sensitization. After nerve injury, nociceptors release excitatory mediators such as substance P and glutamate, which bind to neurokinin 1 (NK1) and N-methyl D-aspartate (NMDA) receptors, respectively, in the dorsal horn. This results in an increase in intracellular calcium concentration and subsequent intracellular activation of the calcium-dependent enzyme protein kinase C (PKC). PKC catalyzes the production of nitric oxide (NO). NO and PKC enhance postsynaptic neuronal excitability by increasing the efficacy of receptor ion channel complexes. The influx of calcium also results in the production of superoxide from mitochondria, with potential cell dysfunction and cell death if intracellular calcium stores are markedly increased for prolonged intervals. COX, cyclooxygenase.

pain, but also of pain from stimuli that are not normally painful (allodynia). For example, a light touch may be described as painful.

Important types of neuropathic pain and their probable causes are shown in Table 1.2, and are discussed in more detail in subsequent chapters.

Pathophysiology. A variety of neuropathic pain syndromes share overlapping pathogenic mechanisms. Those pain syndromes that have unique pathogenic mechanisms are discussed in the relevant chapters. Among other classifications, pathogenic mechanisms can be considered as either peripheral or central.

Peripheral nerve injury produces axonal membrane hyperexcitability that leads to spontaneous generation of ectopic impulses. In addition, changes in the chemical environment surrounding the damaged axon trigger ectopic nerve action potentials, which lead to further impulses (Figure 1.4). Abnormal repetitive firing of injured axons occurs because sodium channels accumulate at the site of injury, creating a lower threshold for the initiation of action potentials (Figure 1.5). Aβ fibers rather than C fibers show the greatest degree of spontaneous ectopic discharge after peripheral nerve injury. Aβ fibers are specialized for light touch and are therefore

TABLE 1.2

Types of neuropathic pain and their probable causes

Type	Cause
Trigeminal neuralgia	Compression of trigeminal ganglion or its branches
Postherpetic neuralgia	Shingles
Complex regional pain syndrome	Trauma/infection/surgery/ inflammation
Diabetic neuropathy	Persistent hyperglycemia (diabetes)
Central pain	Trauma to the spinal cord
	Stroke
Phantom pain	Amputation
Postincisional pain	Surgery

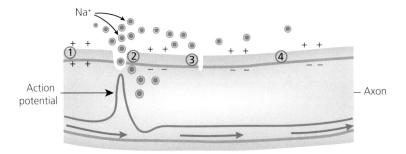

Figure 1.4 Cross-section of an axon, with an action potential (AP) moving from left to right. (1) The AP has passed, the sodium channels are inactivated and the membrane is hyperpolarized. (2) As an impulse passes along the axon the membrane becomes depolarized; at the peak of the AP the sodium channels open and Na+ ions flow into the axon. (3) Na+ ions move in from the adjacent region and depolarize the membrane such that the sodium channels start to open. (4) When the nerve is not transmitting an impulse, a resting potential is maintained across the polarized membrane, with the inside of the axon being negative with respect to the outside.

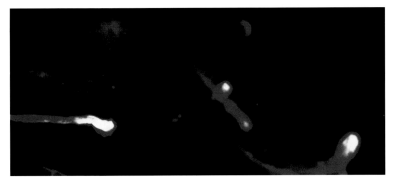

Figure 1.5 Immunofluorescence labeling of sodium channels shows an accumulation of these channels on the membrane of an axon in a chronic neuroma. The intense labeling (yellow) of the end bulbs indicates an increased density and number of sodium channels in the neuroma. This abnormal concentration of sodium channels leads to abnormally persistent repetitive firing of injured nerves. Photograph provided courtesy of Professor M. Devor (Hebrew University of Jerusalem, Israel).

likely to mediate the allodynia experienced after nerve injury. Nerve injury also triggers the production of a series of inflammatory mediators that promote ectopic activity in primary afferent fibers. These mediators are produced by macrophages that migrate to sites of nerve injury and contribute to chronic inflammation in their immediate environment.

Central effects of peripheral nerve injury. The generation of ectopic impulses is not limited to injured axons; neurons of the dorsal root ganglia with damage to the peripheral axons also exhibit spontaneous activity (Figure 1.6). Also, following nerve injury, sympathetic fibers may sprout and form 'baskets' around dorsal root ganglia cell bodies; at the same time, α_2 receptors are produced on neurons of the dorsal root ganglia. These changes allow for activation of the nociceptive neurons via sympathetic fibers.

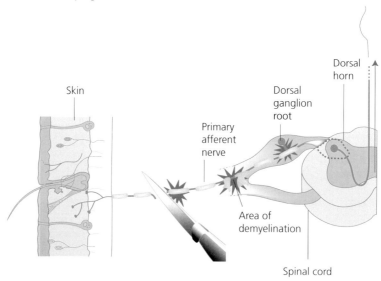

Figure 1.6 Sites of ectopic discharge in damaged primary afferent nociceptors. The regenerating nerve sends out spontaneously active sprouts that are sensitive to mechanical stimuli. A secondary site of hyperactivity develops near the cell body in the dorsal root ganglion (area within dashed line). Ectopic impulses may also arise from a demyelinated section of the primary afferent nociceptor.

More centrally, nerve injury activates NMDA and α-amino-3-hydroxy-5-methyl-4-isoxazole propionic acid (AMPA) receptors. This leads to an increase in intracellular calcium concentration and subsequent intracellular activation of PKC and nitric oxide synthase, with production of NO. NO and PKC enhance postsynaptic neuronal excitability by increasing the efficacy of receptor ion-channel complexes in the postsynaptic membrane. In addition to the activation of NMDA receptors, spinal cord hyperexcitability could be produced by upregulation of sodium channels and voltage-sensitive calcium channels in neurons of the dorsal root ganglia.

The sensitization (increased excitability) and increased synaptic efficacy of second-order neurons termed 'wide dynamic range neurons' (i.e. neurons that respond to a range of noxious and non-noxious stimuli) could explain the allodynia that patients experience after nerve injury. The central hyperexcitable state and enlargement of the area in the periphery where stimulation evokes a neuronal response are sustained by ectopic peripheral nerve activity that causes ongoing release of neurotransmitters in the spinal cord (see Figure 1.3).

Reorganization of neurons. A variety of neuronal growth factors are released after nerve injury; these can produce long-term modifications in neuronal phenotype and in the structural organization of synaptic connectivity through their ability to potentiate over the long term.

Aβ fibers develop abnormal connections with the nociceptive neurons of the dorsal horn. This structural reorganization may underlie the increased sensitivity to normally innocuous mechanical stimulation after nerve injury (Figure 1.7).

In addition, nerve injury triggers glial activation. Glial cells release proinflammatory cytokines (tumor necrosis factor, interleukin-1, interleukin-6) and brain-derived neurotropic factor. These substances, both individually and in concert, contribute to the central hyperexcitability by directly activating neurons (Figure 1.8). Increased glial cell activity normally subsides gradually after injury; its continuation in some patients may be one of the keys to 'what goes wrong in chronic pain'. Chronic use of opioid drugs seems to play a role in glial cell activation, thus increasing pain and decreasing opioid analgesia in a vicious circle (see Figure 1.8).

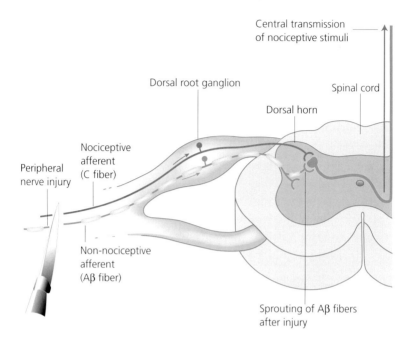

Central transmission
of nociceptive stimuli

Dorsal root ganglion

Spinal cord

Dorsal horn

Nociceptive
afferent
(C fiber)

Peripheral
nerve injury

Non-nociceptive
afferent
(Aβ fiber)

Sprouting of Aβ fibers
after injury

Figure 1.7 Neuronal reorganization and neuropathic pain. Following peripheral nerve injury, persistent pain hypersensitivity may result from new connections between myelinated non-nociceptive Aβ afferent sprouts and nociceptive neurons.

Loss of inhibition. Moreover, after nerve injury there is also a loss of spinal inhibitory control. Mitochondrial superoxide is produced after the influx of calcium associated with nerve injury, and leads to cell dysfunction and the death of interneurons with inhibitory control. The death of these neurons could explain the decrease in GABA, an inhibitory transmitter, in the dorsal horn of the spinal cord after nerve damage, as shown by immunoreactivity experiments (Figure 1.9).

Finally, the persistent afferent input after peripheral nerve injury provokes changes in the nerve structure of the rostroventromedial medulla. These changes in turn encourage tonic discharge (firing at regular intervals) of the descending pathways that facilitate nociceptive transmission, further perpetuating the hyperexcitable state observed after nerve injury.

Genetics and pain

Recent improvements in genetic tools, particularly transgenic knockout mice and microarray-based gene expression profiling, have advanced understanding in this area. In the former, genetic engineering of embryonic stem cell DNA is used to produce a mouse that does not express the target gene. Differences compared with a normal (wild-type) mouse are evaluated: for example, response to different noxious stimuli and to analgesic drugs, revealing six- to tenfold differences in nociceptive and analgesic responses resulting from a single gene manipulation.

In the microarray technique, messenger (m)RNA extracts from tissues of individuals displaying or not displaying nociceptive responses are washed onto a chip that contains DNA probes for thousands of known and unknown genes. Evaluating the degree of mRNA adhesion (hybridization) to the individual DNA probes allows the identification of genes that are expressed differently in the 'pain' versus 'no pain' groups.

Variability in pain response. People report almost ninefold variability in pain intensity in response to a standardized stimulus. This variability is reflected in the degree of activation of 'pain' areas of the brain, such as the anterior cingulate gyrus and somatosensory area 1.

This variation in pain response is reflected in a groundbreaking study of patients with sciatica, in whom a key enzyme (GTP cyclohydrolase 1 [GCH1]) was discovered to be activated and in turn to increase release of the transmitter NO. The marked individual variation in GCH1 activity and NO release correlated with the pain intensity experienced and the risk of developing persistent pain. Identification of a small family of genes that controls the activation of GCH1 and NO release makes it possible that a genetic marker, based on DNA testing, can be developed to determine which patients are at risk of progressing from acute to persistent pain after injury or surgery.

Specific single gene-related abnormalities in pain experience have been identified in humans. Genetic links have been reported for a number of conditions, including hereditary sensory neuropathy type II

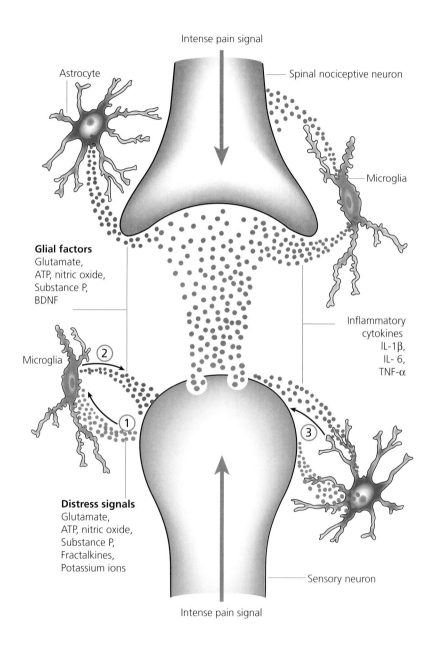

Intense pain signal

Astrocyte

Spinal nociceptive neuron

Microglia

Glial factors
Glutamate,
ATP, nitric oxide,
Substance P,
BDNF

Microglia

Inflammatory
cytokines
IL-1β,
IL- 6,
TNF-α

Distress signals
Glutamate,
ATP, nitric oxide,
Substance P,
Fractalkines,
Potassium ions

Sensory neuron

Intense pain signal

Figure 1.8 Glial cells, the non-neuronal cells in spinal cord and brain, maintain the chemical environment of neurons and deliver the energy to sustain nerve cells. They monitor and regulate the environment by 'mopping up' neurotransmitters released by neurons and release, when necessary, glial factors such as interleukins (tumor necrosis factor [TNF]α) and brain-derived neurotropic factor (BDNF), which aim to restore balance and aid healing (e.g. in the case of an injured nerve). Neurons also become hypersensitive as a result of glial factor release. (1) After nerve injury, intense signals are transmitted along peripheral sensory neurons to the first synapse in the dorsal horn of the spinal cord. Neurotransmitters cross the synapse to activate spinal neurons (see also Figure 1.3). These transmitters are also conveyed to microglia and to astrocytes as 'distress signals'. (2) Glial cells become 'reactive' in the presence of nerve injury, producing 'glial factors' and reducing the uptake of neurotransmitters. This either reduces the usual inhibitory processes acting on neurons or stimulates neurons to become hypersensitive. (3) Glial cells are also activated by neural distress signals, which induce the healing process of inflammation through release of inflammatory cytokines, but also result in neuronal sensitization. These processes (1–3) can become prolonged, lasting past the time of healing and resulting in chronic neuronal hypersensitivity and persisting (chronic) neuropathic pain. Thus, new treatments for chronic neuropathic pain could focus on the cause of the ongoing pain – overactive glia. At least nine anti-glial drugs are currently being evaluated, including: AV411, which inhibits astrocytes; etanercept, which inhibits activation of microglia; the cannabinoid medicine Sativex, which inhibits CB_2 cannabinoid spinal receptors on glia; and minocycline – an antibiotic that inhibits microglia activation. A side benefit of these drugs may be the slowing of the development of tolerance to opioids – glia appear to play a key role in opioid tolerance and withdrawal.

and familial hemiplegic migraine. An even higher level of specificity has been reached with the report of a single (autosomal dominant) gene that controls one of ten sodium channel subtypes, namely $NaV_{1.7}$. Upregulation of $NaV_{1.7}$ results in the human condition erythromelalgia – a burning neuropathic pain in the feet and associated red warm feet.

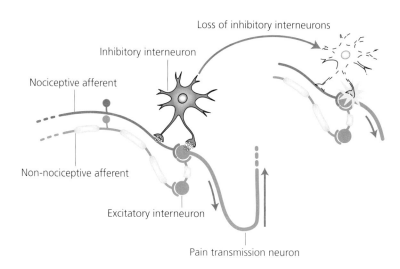

Figure 1.9 Disinhibition and pain. Under normal conditions, inhibitory interneurons actively control sensory inflow. If synthesis of the inhibitory neurotransmitters γ-aminobutyric acid (GABA) and glycine is reduced or the inhibitory interneurons are lost after excessive release of the excitotoxic amino acid glutamate following peripheral nerve injury, the excitability of nociceptive neurons is increased to a level where they begin to respond to normally innocuous inputs. Modified from Scholz & Woolf. *Nat Neurosci* 2002;5:1062–7.

Presumably, the development of $NaV_{1.7}$ blockers will lead to an effective treatment.

Conversely, a surprising discovery is the report of three consanguineous families who exhibited a single (autosomal recessive) gene *SCN9A*, mutations of which caused a loss of function of $NaV_{1.7}$. Individuals with such mutations had a complete congenital inability to experience pain. These findings challenge previous assumptions of substantial neuroplasticity in human pain experience, as $NaV_{1.7}$ seems to be an essential non-redundant requirement for nociception in humans. Also, individuals with the $NaV_{1.7}$ 'channelopathy' have normal sensation (apart from absent nociception) and there is no evidence of neuropathy; they appear to lead normal lives unless they become more likely to attempt dangerous and normally painful feats, such as jumping off a roof. In contrast, the previously identified syndrome of 'congenital insensitivity to pain' is associated with a neuropathy; affected individuals often suffer severe permanent injuries in childhood and may not have normal life expectancy.

It may be of interest in the future to determine whether polymorphisms of *SCN9A* can produce not only the complete inability to experience pain but also interindividual variation in response to a standardized pain stimulus.

Memory and pain

There is strong evidence that learning and memory processes play a key role in determining which patients progress from acute to chronic pain, and continue to experience chronic pain. Such learning processes are accompanied by neuroplasticity changes at multiple levels of the nervous system. Extinction (unlearning) plays a key role in keeping neuroplasticity changes in check after nerve injury. However, in patients with chronic neuropathic pain, extinction processes may be impaired. Training the patient to extinguish pain-related memory processes may be a crucial but difficult key to treatment. Such treatment may be via behavioral, pharmacological or neurostimulation techniques or a combination of these. Innovations in all three of these treatment areas already show promise.

The brain and pain

New sophisticated methods of brain imaging have identified key regions associated with pain and have provided strong evidence that neuroplasticity changes in the brain are associated with chronic pain and accompanying physical dysfunction in humans. A cortical and subcortical network is involved, with the areas most commonly associated being the primary and secondary somatosensory cortices (S_1 and S_2), the anterior cingulated cortex (ACC), the insular cortex (IC), the prefrontal cortex (PFC), the thalamus and, in complex regional pain syndrome, the motor cortex. It is notable that old concepts of a spinothalamic 'pain pathway' provided a very incomplete picture. Also, the involvement of brain areas of the limbic system (e.g. the

ACC and IC) emphasizes the emotional component of human pain experience. In a landmark study by Coghill et al., the degree of unpleasantness associated with pain stimuli correlated closely with activation of the ACC and S_1. This study provided neural correlates of individual differences in the subjective experience of pain. Neuroplasticity changes in the brain have been demonstrated in association with postamputation neuropathic pain, whereby brain representation of an amputated upper limb is 'taken over' by expansion of the area previously representing only the lip area. In patients who have had a spinal cord injury (SCI), the neuroplastic changes are much greater in those who experience pain compared with those with no pain. There is also a correlation between S_1 neuroplastic changes and pain in those who experience pain with the SCI (Figure 1.10). In patients with complex regional pain syndrome, neuroplastic changes in the motor cortex correlate with the motor dysfunction seen in such patients (see Chapter 4). Neuroplastic

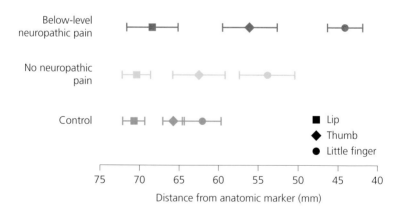

Figure 1.10 Brain neuroplasticity and chronic pain. Distances (in mm) of activated brain regions for lip, thumb and little finger, from a standard brain reference point. Activation by brushing of the skin in the three regions and activation detected in the cortex of the brain (post central gyrus) by functional MRI (fMRI) (mean ± standard error [SE]). Control participants (blue); spinal cord injury (SCI) participants without neuropathic pain (green); SCI participants with neuropathic pain (red).

brain changes probably parallel learning and memory processes. The mechanisms may include: unmasking previously present but inactive synapses; growth of new connections (sprouting), which involves alterations in GABAergic inhibition; and alterations in calcium and sodium channels.

Key points – definitions and mechanisms

- The nervous system is dynamic and plastic; noxious stimuli trigger biological processes that lead to amplification or inhibition of the noxious signal.
- Nociceptive input activates descending pathways that inhibit spinal noxious transmission. These descending pathways are potential targets for analgesic drugs.
- Neuropathic pain is produced by a lesion of the peripheral or central nervous system.
- Nerve injury produces hyperexcitability and spontaneous generation of ectopic impulses in axons and neurons.
- Ectopic peripheral nerve activity contributes to the central hyperexcitable state and the enlargement of neuronal receptive fields.
- After nerve injury there may be a loss of spinal inhibition control resulting from loss of neuronal inhibitory processes, and there may be persistence of glia-induced neuronal hypersensitivity. Both of these maladaptions may play a major role in chronic neuropathic pain.

Key references

Binder A, Baron R. In: Cousins et al., 2009 (see Useful resources).

Blyth FM, March LM, Brnabic AJ et al. Chronic pain in Australia: a prevalence study. *Pain* 2001;89: 127–34.

Brennan F, Carr DB, Cousins M. Pain management: a fundamental human right. *Anesth Analg* 2007;105:205–21.

Coghill RC, McHaffie JG, Yen YF. Neural correlates of interindividual differences in the subjective experience of pain. *Proc Natl Acad Sci USA* 2003;100:8538–42.

Cox JJ, Reimann F, Nicholas AK et al. An SCN9A channelopathy causes congenital inability to experience pain. *Nature* 2006;444:894–8.

Devor M. Neuropathic pain: what do we do with all these theories? *Acta Anaesthesiol Scand* 2001;45:1121–7.

Drenth JP, Waxman SG. Mutations in sodium-channel gene SCN9A cause a spectrum of human genetic pain disorders. *J Clin Invest* 2007;117:3603–9.

Fields RD. New culprits in chronic pain. *Sci Am* 2009;301:50–7.

Hutchinson MR, Coats BD, Lewis SS et al. Proinflammatory cytokines oppose opioid-induced acute and chronic analgesia. *Brain Behav Immun* 2008;22:1178–89.

Melzack R, Wall PD. Pain mechanisms: a new theory. *Science* 1965;150:971–9.

Milligan ED, Watkins LR. Pathological and protective roles of glia in chronic pain. *Nat Rev Neurosci* 2009;10:23–36.

Mogil JS. The genetic mediation of individual differences in sensitivity to pain and its inhibition. *Proc Natl Acad Sci USA* 1999;96:7744–51.

Mogil JS, McCarson KE. Identifying pain genes: bottom-up and top-down approaches. *J Pain* 2000;1:66–80.

National Pain Strategy. National Pain Summit of Australia. www.painsummit.org.au

Siddall PJ, Cousins MJ. Persistent pain as a disease entity: implications for clinical management. *Anesth Analg* 2004;99:510–20.

Siddall PJ, Cousins MJ. In: Cousins et al., 2009 (see Useful resources).

Wrigley PJ, Press SR, Gustin SM et al. Neuropathic pain and primary somatosensory cortex reorganization following spinal cord injury. *Pain* 2009;141:52–9.

The initial evaluation of a patient's pain forms the foundation for a rational treatment plan and so it must be as thorough as possible. For patients with chronic pain, this evaluation should include:

- a general medical history, including a detailed pain history (see Table 2.1)
- a physical examination (paying particular attention to neurological and musculoskeletal function)
- a psychosocial assessment
- diagnostic testing (e.g. imaging), when appropriate.

Clearly, the history, physical examination and any laboratory evaluation performed to assess chronic pain may overlap with those carried out for general medical diagnosis and therapy.

Many patients with pain due to cancer or other serious illnesses such as HIV/AIDS experience pain from multiple mechanisms, locations and etiologies (see Chapter 8, Table 8.1). These patients may simultaneously experience: acute and chronic pain; somatic and neuropathic pain related to the primary diagnosis or its treatment; or pain from unrelated, possibly pre-existing, medical conditions.

Because of the multiple and evolving etiologies of pain, each time a clinician assesses any patient at risk of undertreated pain, there must be a fresh evaluation of the pain. Unless pain is assessed systematically and classified according to its likely origin as well as its temporal pattern, aggravating and ameliorating factors and perpetuating factors and comorbidities, then the patient is at risk of receiving suboptimal treatment. Even after an initial pain treatment plan is put in place, the source and severity of a person's pain and the effectiveness of treatment may fluctuate, and therefore their pain should be reviewed and documented at regular intervals. The patient is a key partner in this.

History

The patient's pain history should document details concerning the circumstances surrounding the beginning of the episode to ascertain

TABLE 2.1

Areas to explore when taking the patient's pain history

- Brief overview of pain site(s)
- History of present illness: include detailed history of current pain
- Past and concurrent medical/surgical history
  - prior patient submission of 'time line' (i.e. the chronological sequence of medical and surgical conditions and treatments)
  - highlight significant issues for current pain/treatment
- Family history: highlight chronic pain problems
- Medication (past and present)
  - dose/duration, effectiveness, side effects
  - alcohol, substances, smoking, other
- Other treatments used and healthcare professionals consulted
- Imaging and other investigations
- Psychosocial history
- Review of systems

Detailed current pain history

- Circumstances associated with pain onset
- Primary site of pain (use of pain diagram)

- Radiation of pain
- Character of pain (using McGill Melzack Multidimensional Pain Inventory [e.g. is pain throbbing, sharp, aching?])
- Intensity of pain (e.g. on visual analog scale)
  - at rest
  - on movement
  - at present
  - during last week
  - highest level
- Factors altering pain
  - what makes pain worse?
  - what makes it better?
- Associated symptoms (e.g. nausea)
- Temporal factors
  - is pain present continuously or otherwise?
  - are there paroxysmal episodes?
- Effect of pain on sleep
- Effect of pain on work and activities of daily living
- Effect of pain on social and recreational activities
- Effect of pain on mood
- Expectations of outcome of pain treatment

CONTINUED

TABLE 2.1 (CONTINUED)

- Patient's belief concerning the causes of pain
- Reduction in pain required to resume 'reasonable activities'
- Patient's typical coping response for stress or pain
- Family expectations and beliefs about pain, stress and disease
- Ways the patient describes or shows pain
- Patient's knowledge, expectations and preferences for pain management

Adapted from Vije and Ashburn, 2009.

biomechanical and other physical forces that heighten the risk for specific injuries. For example, lifting and twisting causing lower spinal or shoulder injury, repetitive motion causing tendonitis, a fall from a height causing spinal fracture or a motor vehicle accident causing cervical, brachial plexus or traumatic brain injury. Aspects such as the location, duration, type and intensity of the pain, exacerbating or alleviating factors, previous treatments and response to them, and the meaning of the pain to the patient and their family should also be recorded in detail (Table 2.1).

The patient's self-report is a more accurate assessment of pain than vital signs, outward behavior or observer estimates; however, the last is, by default, important in neonates, infants and individuals of any age with severe cognitive impairment or poor language skills. To avoid underestimating pain in individuals with poor cognition or in those incapable of communicating, indirect indices of pain such as facial expression or body language become more important.

Pain location. It is helpful to ask patients to identify on a body map the areas where they experience pain (Figure 2.1). Body pain maps may help classify pain, as in the case of peripheral neuropathic pain with different causes (see Chapter 5).

Pain radiation. Identification of pain radiation, where present, may be of assistance in evaluating possible source of pain (e.g. pain from a

Patient Name: _____

Date: _____

Clinician Name: _____

1. Indicate (in blue ink) on the figures below area(s) of consistent pain.

2. Indicate (in red ink) on the figures below area(s) of intermittent chronic pain.

3. Indicate level of pain on the scale below.

0	1	2	3	4	5	6	7	8	9	10

no pain   worst imaginable pain

4. Describe how the above indicated pain affects your functioning:

_____

_____

_____

5. Other: _____

Clinician: _____

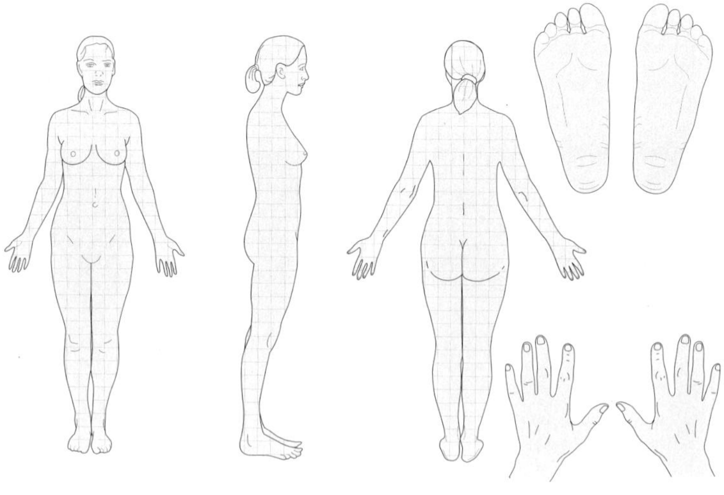

Figure 2.1 Pain assessment form, including a body map, which can be used to document pain symptoms such as location and intensity.

compressed spinal nerve may radiate down the leg to the foot or down the arm to the hand).

Pain character may help to differentiate somatic, visceral and neuropathic pain. Neuropathic pain can be diagnosed more accurately if a validated instrument is used as illustrated by Table 2.2.

Pain intensity is the most frequently evaluated dimension of pain. During the titration of analgesics for acute time-limited pain of obvious cause (e.g. dental extraction), it may suffice to monitor only pain intensity and forego tracking of other aspects of the multidimensional pain experience.

Assessment tools. Three types of assessment tool are commonly used to quantify pain intensity (Figure 2.2): visual analog scale (VAS); numeric rating scale (NRS); and adjective rating scale (ARS). The VAS is presented graphically with a 10-cm line and endpoint descriptors. Patients place a mark on the line at a point that best represents their pain. Their responses are scored by measuring the distance of the

TABLE 2.2

Screening tools for neuropathic pain

Items	S-LANSS	painDETECT
Pricking, tingling	+	+
Electric shocks or shooting	+	+
Hot or burning	+	+
Numbness	−	+
Pain evoked by light touch	+	+
Other symptoms	Autonomic changes	Temporal and referred patterns
Clinical examination	Brush allodynia Raised pinprick threshold	Pain evoked by hot/cold stimuli

painDETECT, questionnaire designed to identify neuropathic components in patients with back pain; S-LANSS, self-report version of the Leeds Assessment of Neuropathic Symptoms and Signs pain scale.
Adapted from Bennett et al., *Pain* 2007;127:199–203.

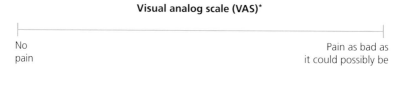

Visual analog scale (VAS)*

No pain — Pain as bad as it could possibly be

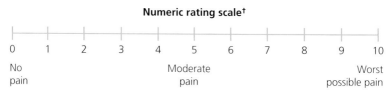

Numeric rating scale†

0 1 2 3 4 5 6 7 8 9 10

No pain — Moderate pain — Worst possible pain

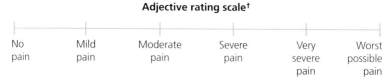

Adjective rating scale†

No pain — Mild pain — Moderate pain — Severe pain — Very severe pain — Worst possible pain

*A 10-cm baseline is recommended for VAS.
†If used as a graphic rating scale, a 10-cm baseline is recommended.

Figure 2.2 Pain intensity scales.

mark from the leftmost end of the scale (the 'anchor'). This scale is used primarily in research studies.

The NRS may be presented graphically or verbally, with 0 representing 'no pain' and 10 representing 'the worst possible pain'. Patients volunteer a number that best represents their pain intensity. A change of two points on the scale is clinically meaningful.

The ARS employs descriptors of pain intensity such as 'none', 'mild', 'moderate' or 'severe'.

Clinicians often anchor the numerical scale numbers with adjectives denoting levels of both pain intensity and function, giving the numbers consensual meaning between patient and clinician.

Patient's perception. We now know that the decrement in pain intensity experienced by an individual relates to that patient's baseline (pretreatment) pain intensity. The more severe the baseline pain, the greater the decrement in VAS or NRS score needed to achieve clinical importance for the patient.

Examination

It is essential to perform comprehensive neurological and musculoskeletal examinations in addition to other routine physical assessment. The neurological examination should evaluate:

- mental status
- motor system
- sensory perception
- deep tendon reflexes
- cranial nerve function.

Mental status. An evaluation of mental status should assess the items listed in Table 2.3. The patient may be asked to remember several objects mentioned earlier in the course of the examination, to repeat sentences, to solve simple mathematical problems or to carry out commands of graded complexity. In the case of depressed mood, the clinician should enquire about suicidal ideation, because of the increased risk associated with chronic pain.

Motor system. An evaluation of the motor system should check the appearance of the muscles (e.g. atrophy), their tone (e.g. flaccid, taut, tender) and strength. Observation of gait can provide information on muscle strength; any indication of impaired vestibular, cerebellar or

TABLE 2.3

Items for assessment in the evaluation of mental status

- Level of alertness
- Degree of orientation with respect to time, place and person
- General appearance
- Behavior and mood

- Intellectual function, including:
  - comprehension
  - ability to pay attention
  - insight
  - memory

dorsal column function should be documented. Latent weakness can be detected by asking patients to walk on their toes and heels. Heel walking is the most sensitive bedside test for weakness of foot dorsiflexion, while toe walking is the best way to detect early weakness of foot plantar flexion.

Muscle atrophy can be documented by circumferential measurements of the extremities (e.g. the calf and thigh bilaterally). A difference of 2 cm or more at the same level is indicative of atrophy.

Sensory perception can be evaluated with different types of stimuli, such as light touch, painful squeeze or pinprick, temperature and pressure/vibration. A freshly opened alcohol wipe may be used as a bedside probe of deficits in cold perception or to elicit cold allodynia.

Deep tendon reflex testing is the most objective part of the neurological examination, as the reflexes are not under voluntary control and testing does not depend on the patient's cooperation. Alterations in reflexes are often early signs of neurological dysfunction.

Pathological reflexes, such as Babinski (foot) and Hoffmann (hand) indicating upper motor neuron dysfunction (e.g. spinal cord compression), should be tested.

Cranial nerve function. The 12 cranial nerves relay messages between the brain and the head and neck. They mediate motor and sensory functions, including vision, smell and movement of the tongue and vocal cords. The evaluation of the fifth cranial nerve (affected in trigeminal neuralgia, see Chapter 3) requires the assessment of facial sensation, jaw strength and movement, and corneal reflexes.

Musculoskeletal examination is important for all patients because of secondary pain related to postural changes, and deconditioning resulting in muscle atrophy, as well as the adoption of abnormal patterns of movement and loss of range of movement in the spine and various joints. All of these can result in a vicious circle of loss of function and increasing pain, as well as a potential for tropic changes. Additionally, certain pain conditions originate in a particular primary musculoskeletal site (e.g. the lumbar spine or other joints). Even in these patients secondary musculoskeletal changes should be sought. Details of what to include in the general and specific examinations are listed in Table 2.4.

Psychosocial assessment

The psychosocial assessment should explore the patient's:

- mood
- coping skills
- family support structure
- signs and symptoms of anxiety, depression and sleep disorder
- expectations regarding pain management.

Persistent pain commonly undermines mood, sleep, vitality, function and other dimensions of health-related quality of life (HRQoL). Thus, it is important to monitor how pain and its treatment affect function, daily activities, mood, sleep patterns and other aspects of HRQoL. Scales such as the Brief Pain Inventory, which evaluates pain intensity and the effect of pain on mood, sleep, social function and activities, are commonly used to monitor the effects of treatment from visit to visit.

Quality-of-life questionnaires specifically designed for patients with chronic non-malignant pain have been developed in an effort to better gauge how pain and pain treatments affect HRQoL. For example, the Treatment Outcomes in Pain Survey (TOPS) is a 61-item questionnaire (Table 2.5) that augments the SF-36 Medical Outcomes Study with items originally adapted from the Multidimensional Pain Inventory and the Oswestry Disability Questionnaire. The TOPS is validated in cancer and various chronic pain populations.

Assessment for risk of substance abuse

As noted in Chapter 1, glial activation and other neuroplastic changes in chronic pain underlie a gradual decline in the effectiveness of opioid analgesics (tolerance), leading to dose escalation and reduced duration

TABLE 2.4

Items for inclusion in the physical examination

General examination*

- Observation of posture when sitting, standing, lying and 'at rest'
- Bilateral knee raise
- Squat and rise
- Areas of muscle spasm or trigger points

Specific examination

- All major joints, noting active, passive and resisted range of movement and any local pain on palpation
- Shoulders, particularly, to detect inflammatory or adhesive capsulitis[†] and to examine for brachial plexopathy causing radicular pain down the arm into the hand
- Elbows, for signs of ligamentous or tendonous inflammation
- Wrists, for signs of carpal or ulnar tunnel syndrome
- Knees, for signs of abnormal patellar tracking
- Hips, for signs of trochanteric bursitis
- Ankles and feet for postural abnormalities or plantar fasciitis

Detailed spine examination

- Signs of scoliosis, kyphosis, pelvic tilt
- Palpate midline for tenderness over spinous processes (vertebral bodies) and disks, and paravertebrally for facet tenderness
- Flexion, extension, lateral flexion, rotation
  - pain on flexion may point to muscle spasm
  - pain on extension/rotation or ipsilateral pain on lateral flexion may point to facet-related pain (may also be pain on palpation paravertebrally)
- Sacroiliac joint (SIJ) palpation may be positive in presence of inflammation; various tests of SIJ movement can be helpful
  - straight-leg raising or sitting leg extension that elicits pain radiating to the foot or in the contralateral low back may indicate lumbosacral nerve root irritation or compression from lumbar disk protrusion or spinal stenosis[‡]

CONTINUED

TABLE 2.4 (CONTINUED)

Other examinations

- Routinely check blood pressure, pulse, respiratory rate and temperature

- Detailed examination of other body systems depends on patient's history, for example:

  – peripheral vascular system for limb pain

  – thorax and abdomen for abdominal pain

  – abdomen and distal pulses for patients > 50 years with lumbar pain, to check for an abdominal aortic aneurysm

*Should build on any findings from the neurological examination of the motor system.
†Common with deconditioning.
‡Often tested in neurological examination.

of analgesic effects. Some patients may become anxious about loss of efficiency and may exhibit symptoms and signs resembling addiction ('pseudo-addiction'). Others may develop behaviors that satisfy all the criteria for addiction. Recently it has been recognized that there is a spectrum of responses that require assessment of 'risk of substance abuse' in each patient using opioids, benzodiazepines or other medications associated with dependence. This assessment needs to be carried out before starting such medications and at intervals during treatment. A number of instruments are now available to assess the level of risk for aberrant medication-related behavior.

Diagnostic tests

Imaging tests can help physicians confirm or rule out diagnoses suggested by findings in the medical history or physical examination. Radiographs provide details of bone structure, while bone scans are performed to rule out occult fractures (small fractures not visible on routine radiographs) or inflammatory processes (such as infection or certain tumors). Bone scans also help determine whether a compression fracture of the vertebral body is old or new, as an old

TABLE 2.5

Example questions taken from the Treatment Outcomes in Pain Survey

1. The following items concern activities you might perform during a typical day. Does your health now limit you in these activities? If so, by how much?

	Not at all	A little	A lot
Vigorous activities (e.g. running, lifting heavy objects, participating in strenuous sports)			
Moderate activities (e.g. moving a table, pushing a vacuum cleaner, bowling or playing golf)			
Climbing several flights of stairs			
Climbing one flight of stairs			
Bending, kneeling or stooping			
Walking more than a mile			
Walking several blocks			
Walking one block			
Bathing or dressing yourself			
Combing your hair			
Writing			
Talking			

2. During the past 4 weeks, to what extent has your physical health or emotional problems interfered with your normal social activities with family, friends, neighbors or groups?

Not at all   Slightly   Moderately   Quite a bit   Extremely

3. How much does your pain get in the way of:

	Not at all	A little	Moderately	Quite a lot	A lot
Enjoying your social activities or hobbies?					
Doing any social activities or hobbies?					
Getting along with your husband/wife/ significant other/family?					
Getting along with friends outside of your family?					
The pleasure you get from being with your family?					
How well you can plan things?					

fracture will not 'light up', but a new one will. However, they cannot differentiate between tumor, infection or fracture with adjoining inflammation. In such cases, CT or MRI can better characterize the lesion.

Similarly, in patients whose findings suggest nerve impairment, CT or MRI can help define a possible anatomic cause. However, there is no 1:1 relationship between imaging findings and pain. Indeed, severe degenerative changes may be present with no accompanying pain and vice versa. Imaging studies are therefore no substitute for careful history taking and physical examination.

Key points – assessment of pain

- A thorough evaluation of pain history and a detailed examination are the foundations for a rational treatment plan.
- Persistent pain is a disease entity per se that can undermine many dimensions of health-related quality of life.
- The patient's pain history should document the onset, location, radiation, duration, type (character) and intensity of pain, exacerbating or alleviating factors, previous treatments and response to them, and the meaning of the pain to the patient and their family.
- Assessment of patients with chronic pain should include a physical examination with particular attention to neurological and musculoskeletal function, a psychosocial assessment and, when appropriate, diagnostic testing such as imaging.

Key references

Ballantyne JC, LaForge KS. Opioid dependence and addiction during opioid treatment of chronic pain. *Pain* 2007;129:235–55.

Bennett MI, Attal N, Backonja MM et al. Using screening tools to identify neuropathic pain. *Pain* 2007;127:199–203.

Blyth FM, Macfarlane GJ, Nicholas MK. The contribution of psychosocial factors to the development of chronic pain: the key to better outcomes for patients? *Pain* 2007;129:8–11.

Butler SF, Budman SH, Fernandez KC et al. Development and validation of the Current Opioid Misuse Measure. *Pain* 2007;130:144–56.

Nicholas MK, Asghari A, Blyth FM. What do the numbers mean? Normative data in chronic pain measures. *Pain* 2008;134:158–73.

Rogers WH, Wittink HM, Ashburn MA et al. Using the "TOPS," an outcomes instrument for multidisciplinary outpatient pain treatment. *Pain Med* 2000;1:55–67.

Turk DC, Dworkin RH, Burke LB et al. Developing patient-reported outcome measures for pain clinical trials: IMMPACT recommendations. *Pain* 2006;125:208–15.

Vije C, Ashburn MA. In: Cousins et al., 2009 (see Useful resources).

Trigeminal neuralgia is an idiopathic paroxysmal recurrent pain in the distribution of one or more branches of the trigeminal (fifth cranial) nerve (Figure 3.1).

Pathophysiology

Pain is thought to be caused by vascular compression of the trigeminal ganglion or its branches (Figure 3.2), but bony abnormalities or otherwise inapparent multiple sclerosis (MS) could also be contributors. Surveys of MS clinics have shown that 2% of patients with MS have trigeminal neuralgia; furthermore, in 0.2% of these patients trigeminal neuralgia was diagnosed before MS was diagnosed. Rarely, a space-occupying lesion (e.g. tumor) in the cerebellopontine angle can be a

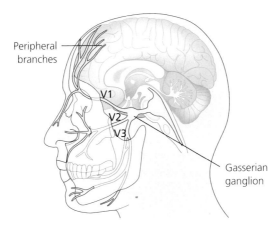

Figure 3.1 Location and structure of the trigeminal nerve. It has three branches (or divisions): the upper first branch (ophthalmic; V1), which runs above the eye, forehead and front of the head; the middle second branch (maxillary; V2), which runs through the cheek, upper jaw, teeth and gums, and side of the nose; and the lower third branch (mandibular; V3), which runs through the lower jaw, teeth and gums. All three branches meet at the Gasserian ganglion.

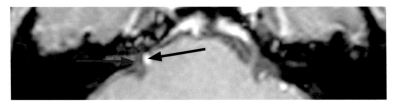

Figure 3.2 Magnetic resonance image showing vascular compression of the trigeminal ganglion in a patient with trigeminal neuralgia. The red arrow points to the right trigeminal nerve (gray area); the black arrow points to the vascular loop (branch of the posteroinferior cerebellar artery; white area).

cause of trigeminal neuralgia, particularly if there is loss of sensation in trigeminal territory – sometimes called atypical trigeminal neuralgia.

Compression of the peripheral branches of the trigeminal nerve can also occur intraorally or in the region of the chin as the result of trauma, metastatic tumor or injury during alveolar or mandibular bone excision during tooth extraction.

About 5% of people with trigeminal neuralgia have other family members with the disorder, which suggests a possible genetic cause in some cases.

Injury to the nerve root renders axons and axotomized neurons in the Gasserian ganglion hyperexcitable. A discharge from the Gasserian ganglion is then thought to spread to neighboring neurons, triggering them to fire in turn. Therefore, although trigeminal neuralgia may have an initially inapparent peripheral origin, the clinical syndrome results from abnormal discharges within clusters of central neurons in the trigeminal nucleus and/or abnormal central processing of afferent neural impulses.

Diagnosis

Because there are no objective tests for trigeminal neuralgia, clinical manifestations are the mainstay of diagnosis. Trigeminal neuralgia is more prevalent in women than men by a ratio of 3:2. It can occur at any age, but usually has its onset in individuals over 50 years old.

Clinical features. Trigeminal neuralgia is characterized by paroxysmal and recurrent attacks of facial pain that are sudden and unilateral, and that follow the distribution of one or more divisions of the trigeminal nerve. Pain is precipitated from trigger areas or by innocuous daily activities such as eating, talking, washing the face or brushing the teeth. Patients are asymptomatic between paroxysms. The pain is often severe. Patients describe it as sharp, stabbing or burning in quality, usually lasting between a few seconds and less than 2 minutes. Despite the brief duration of paroxysms, patients become terrified of each paroxysm because of the severity and unpredictability.

Differential diagnosis. Other diagnoses should be considered if the pain is bilateral or continuous and if there are no evident provoking factors, such as idiopathic (atypical) facial pain, muscular pain, dental pain or one of the headache syndromes (e.g. cluster headache or migraine). If there are ocular disturbances, systemic symptoms (e.g. fever, anorexia or weight loss) and tenderness to palpation of the temporal area, temporal arteritis should be considered. Temporal arteritis is a key diagnosis because it can lead to blindness if treatment is delayed. Rarely, a combination of trigeminal neuralgia and cluster headache may occur (cluster tic) (see Chapter 11).

Imaging. The most important diagnostic imaging technique is MRI. MRI can identify benign or malignant lesions or plaques of MS. In addition, high-resolution MRI (e.g. three-dimensional fast-inflow MRI with steady-state precession) now enables a much more detailed study of the trigeminal nerve and its spatial relation with vascular structures such as a vascular loop (see Figure 3.2).

Management

Pharmacological management. Meta-analyses of randomized controlled trials show the anticonvulsant sodium channel blocker carbamazepine, 800–1200 mg/day, to be effective. In general, one in every three individuals receiving carbamazepine will experience pain relief. Frequent adverse events include sedation and dizziness. Rare adverse events are decreased platelet or white blood cell counts and, in the older age group, sodium retention.

Lamotrigine, a sodium channel blocker, slowly titrated to reach 100–400 mg/day, may have an additional effect in patients who obtain insufficient relief with carbamazepine. Other options include the gabapentinoids (gabapentin or pregabalin), particularly in older people or in patients who are unable to tolerate carbamazepine. Pregabalin has an advantage because the dose can be more rapidly titrated than the gabapentin dose, and both gabapentinoids have a lower side effect burden than either carbamazepine or lamotrigine.

In patients with unresponsive pain, it may be necessary to use a systemic infusion of lidocaine (lignocaine), aiming for a blood concentration of 1–2 µg/mL. In adults this usually requires infusion of 50–100 mg/hour (0.5–1.0 mL/hour of 10% lidocaine) delivered via a subcutaneous needle or cannula.

Invasive procedures

If medical management has failed and the patient can tolerate surgery, microvascular decompression of the trigeminal neural complex is the preferred treatment. This procedure directly treats the cause of the problem without destroying any neural tissue. Morbidity and mortality are low. Pain relief persists in more than 85% of patients at 5-year follow-up, with no risk of sensory loss. Many patients have complete abolition of pain – a result that is attainable for very few chronic pain conditions.

In older patients, percutaneous radiofrequency lesioning of the affected components of the trigeminal complex is the method of choice. This is a rapid and highly controllable procedure that aims to minimize risk of sensory loss. However, pain tends to recur after about 3 years and about 5% of patients have painful sensory loss (anesthesia dolorosa).

Balloon compression and retro-Gasserian glycerol injection are alternative lesioning procedures. Unfortunately, there are no comparative studies among invasive procedures, so the choice is often guided by operator expertise in a particular technique.

For non-responders and those in whom the pain relief is only temporary, a new or repeat procedure is sometimes performed. The long-term effectiveness of this strategy is unknown, and the risk of producing new neurological deficits is higher. Patients who elect to undergo repeat procedures should be informed of the increased risks.

Because of the severity and unpredictability of episodes of trigeminal neuralgia, patients with ineffective treatment pain are at increased risk of suicide. Risk of suicide is discussed in *Fast Facts: Depression*.

Key points – trigeminal neuralgia

- Trigeminal neuralgia is characterized by paroxysmal and recurrent attacks of facial pain that are sudden and unilateral, and follow the distribution of one or more divisions of the trigeminal nerve.
- Pain is caused by compression of the trigeminal ganglion or its branches.
- Medical management remains the first line of treatment. Carbamazepine, traditionally the drug of choice, is being replaced by gabapentin and pregabalin because of fewer side effects.
- Failed medical treatment is an indication for consideration of mircovascular decompression or alternative techniques.

Key references

Devor M, Amir R, Rappaport ZH. Pathophysiology of trigeminal neuralgia: the ignition hypothesis. *Clin J Pain* 2002;18:4–13.

Haddad M, Gunn J. *Fast Facts: Depression*, 3rd edn. Oxford: Health Press Limited, 2011.

Peters G, Nurmikko TJ. Peripheral and gasserian ganglion-level procedures for the treatment of trigeminal neuralgia. *Clin J Pain* 2002;18:28–34.

Rappaport ZH, Devor M. TIC and cranial neuralgias In: Schmidt RF, Willis WD, eds. *Encyclopedia of Pain*. Heidelberg: Springer, 2007: 2482–5.

Sindrup SH, Jensen TS. Pharmacotherapy of trigeminal neuralgia. *Clin J Pain* 2002;18:22–7.

Zakrzewska JM. Diagnosis and differential diagnosis of trigeminal neuralgia. *Clin J Pain* 2002;18: 14–21.

The term 'complex regional pain syndrome' (CRPS) was coined in 1995 by the International Association for the Study of Pain (IASP) to replace terms previously used to describe the condition. The diagnosis of CRPS requires the presence of several factors, which may include sensory, vascular and motor abnormalities as well as edema and sweating abnormalities. The syndrome encompasses an array of painful conditions characterized by continuing (spontaneous and/or evoked) regional pain that is seemingly disproportionate in time or degree to the usual course of any known trauma or other lesion. The pain is regional (that is, not in a specific nerve territory or dermatome) and usually has a distal predominance of abnormal sensory, motor, sudomotor, vasomotor and/or trophic findings. The syndrome shows variable progression over time. Harden et al. have published statistically derived criteria (the 'Budapest criteria') for clinical diagnosis (see Table 4.1). More information on diagnosis is also available from the IASP (www.iasp-pain.org; see Table 4.2).

A conservative estimate of the combined incidence of CRPS types I and II is 6 new cases per 100 000 person years at risk and a prevalence of about 21 per 100 000 people. CRPS type I, previously called 'reflex sympathetic dystrophy', in which there is no definable lesion, develops more often than CRPS type II, previously called 'causalgia', in which there is a defined nerve lesion. The incidence of CRPS II in peripheral nerve injury varies from 2% to 14% in different studies, with a mean of 4%. The incidence of CRPS I is 1–2% after fractures, 12% after brain lesions, 5% after myocardial infarction and 0.7% after total knee replacement surgery.

Pathophysiology

CRPS may be triggered by a variety of events, such as trauma, surgery, inflammatory processes, cerebrovascular accidents and nerve injury. No precipitating factor can be identified in approximately 10% of cases.

TABLE 4.1

'Budapest criteria' for diagnosis of CRPS

The following criteria must be met for a clinical diagnosis

- Continuing pain, which is disproportionate to any inciting event
- Must report at least one symptom in **three of the four** following categories:
  - sensory: reports of hyperesthesia and/or allodynia
  - vasomotor: reports of temperature asymmetry and/or skin color changes and/or skin color asymmetry
  - sudomotor/edema: reports of edema and/or sweating changes and/or sweating asymmetry
  - motor/trophic: reports of decreased range of motion and/or motor dysfunction (weakness, tremor, dystonia) and/or trophic changes (hair, nail, skin)
- Must display at least **one sign** at the time of evaluation in **two or more** of the following categories
  - sensory: evidence of hyperalgesia (to pinprick) and/or allodynia (to light touch and/or temperature sensation and/or deep somatic pressure and/or joint movement)
  - vasomotor: evidence of temperature asymmetry (> 1°C) and/or skin color changes and/or asymmetry
  - sudomotor/edema: evidence of edema and/or sweating changes and/or sweating asymmetry
  - motor/trophic: evidence of decreased range of motion and/or motor dysfunction (weakness, tremor, dystonia) and/or trophic changes (hair, nail, skin)
- There is no other diagnosis that better explains the signs and symptoms

From Harden et al., 2007.

After some initial controversy, psychological factors are now no longer viewed as etiologic contributors (see 'Psychological processes', page 51). In addition to the pathogenic mechanisms common to all types of neuropathic pain, there are some features that are particularly 47

TABLE 4.2

Diagnostic criteria for complex regional pain syndrome*

Clinical signs/symptoms

Positive sensory abnormalities

- Spontaneous pain
- Mechanical hyperalgesia
- Thermal hyperalgesia
- Deep somatic hyperalgesia

Vascular abnormalities

- Vasodilation
- Vasoconstriction
- Skin temperature asymmetries[†]
- Skin color changes[†]

Edema, sweating abnormalities

- Swelling
- Hyperhidrosis
- Hypohidrosis

Motor trophic changes

- Motor weakness
- Tremor
- Dystonia
- Coordination deficits
- Nail, hair changes
- Skin atrophy
- Joint stiffness
- Soft tissue changes

Interpretation for clinical use

≥ 1 symptoms from ≥ 3 categories each and ≥ 1 signs of ≥ 2 categories each; sensitivity 0.85; specificity 0.60

*From the International Association for the Study of Pain (www.iasp-pain.org).
[†] See Figure 4.1.

characteristic of CRPS. Animal studies have shown that nerve injury is followed by:
- sprouting of noradrenergic axons around sensory neurons at the corresponding dorsal root ganglia
- upregulation of α_2-adrenoreceptors
- an abnormally intense response of injured axons to sympathetic stimulation.

The abnormal innervation and excitation by sympathetic stimulation provide a possible explanation for the abnormal discharges in peripheral nerves that are observed following nerve damage as well as the reactivity of pain to psychological distress.

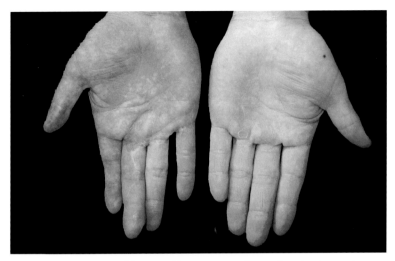

Figure 4.1 A 23-year-old man with type I complex regional pain syndrome. He had a 1-year history of pain in his right hand following direct trauma. He presented with edema and changes in temperature and skin color. The right hand is reddish, with muscle atrophy.

In humans, the nature and extent of involvement of the sympathetic nervous system is less clear (see below). Pain alleviation after sympathetic nerve blockade or sympatholytic drug therapy is not consistent, and relapses are common.

Motor abnormalities, found in 50% of CRPS patients, are most probably generated by changes in brain motor neurons. Baron's group in Germany has reported disturbed integration of visual and proprioceptive inputs in the posterior parietal cortices of CRPS patients. Also, functional MRI during finger tapping of the affected limb in CRPS patients showed reorganization of central motor circuits. The degree of reorganization correlated with the extent of motor dysfunction detected by clinical examination. Thus, it seems clear that maladaptive changes in the brain motor system contribute to motor symptoms in patients with CRPS. This is further evidence of chronic pain as a 'disease entity'. Behavioral/physical treatments aimed at motor components of CRPS in the brain have been described as 'reprogramming the brain'.

49

Immune-cell-mediated inflammation and cytokine release. Skin biopsies in the affected limbs of patients with CRPS show evidence of ongoing inflammation. Proinflammatory cytokines and high levels of interleukin (IL)-6 and tumor necrosis factor (TNF)α, as well as tryptase (a measure of mast cell activity), occur in the fluid of artificially produced skin blisters. Also, CRPS patients with skin hyperalgesia, have been found to have higher levels of soluble TNFα receptor type-1 than patients without hyperalgesia, again indicating a role for peripheral inflammation.

The patchy osteoporosis in advanced CRPS may reflect regional inflammation in deep somatic tissues, as both IL-1 and IL-6 cause proliferation and activation of osteoclasts (bone resorption) and suppress activity of osteoblasts (bone deposition). There is also some evidence of an autoimmune response in patients with CRPS – possibly triggered by infection with *Campylobacter* spp.

However, all of the above peripheral processes do not explain more central phenomena, such as motor abnormalities in the brain, or response to spinal cord stimulation and epidural clonidine (see page 55).

Sympathetically maintained pain (SMP) refers to a subset of CRPS patients whose pain is relieved (at least on a temporary basis) by a correctly applied sympatholytic intervention. Those who do not respond are deemed to have sympathetically independent pain (SIP).

Studies in humans by Baron's group now confirm that in both CRPS I and II, cutaneous nociceptors develop catecholamine sensitivity. This appears to occur through a coupling between sympathetic noradrenergic neurons and primary afferent nociceptors at the peripheral level. The actual mechanism of the linkage is different in CRPS I compared with CRPS II. The nerve injury in CRPS II results in coupling at the level of the nerve lesion and also at the dorsal root ganglion. The evidence is less clear for CRPS I. However, it appears that coupling occurs at skin level and in deep somatic tissues.

The pain-relieving effects of sympathetic blocks in patients with SMP outlast the conduction block of sympathetic neurons – in a small number of cases producing permanent relief if applied early in the course of CRPS. It appears that, in SMP, spinal cord sympathetic neurons maintain a positive feedback via sympathetic efferents and then primary afferent nociceptors. Sympathetic block switches off the sympathetic chain, decreases sensitization of afferent nociceptors which, in turn, decreases input to spinal afferents and then to spinal sympathetic neurons. Unfortunately, in most patients, spinal hyperactivity resumes when the block wears off.

The percentage of pain that depends on sympathetic activity declines during the course of CRPS. After about 2 years, there is only a small chance that sympatholytic interventions might be successful.

Psychological processes. There is general agreement that CRPS is associated with emotional and behavioral distress, as might be expected when a person suffers from an extremely painful and often disabling condition with an uncertain prospect for helpful treatment, and often stigmatization. As with most patients with neuropathic pain conditions, psychological distress activates the sympathetic system, and this accounts for the worsening of CRPS pain. There is no evidence of a 'CRPS personality'. The psychological symptoms and psychiatric comorbidities observed in patients with CRPS have a similar distribution in patients with other chronic pain syndromes, supporting the idea that psychological dysfunction is the result of prolonged pain and disability and not the cause of the syndrome itself.

Diagnostic tests

A number of diagnostic tests have been evaluated in patients with CRPS, but diagnosis of the condition remains a clinical one (see Tables 4.1 and 4.2). Radiological abnormalities such as cortical thinning and cortical bone loss (due to increased osteoclastic activity) are often present in CRPS. Patients with CRPS have an abnormal third phase of bone scintigraphy, which is characterized by increased periarticular uptake involving multiple joints in the affected extremity. However, a critical review of bone scintigraphy in the diagnosis of CRPS reported wide variability in scintigraphic changes, with very low sensitivity and specificity. Loss of functional use due to splinting and guarding and changes in regional blood flow could explain the imaging findings.

Treatment

A lack of understanding of pathophysiological abnormalities, and differing views on diagnostic criteria, has hampered the selection of well-defined populations of CRPS patients to participate in controlled trials of potential treatments. Three literature reviews found little consistent information, and consequently the treatment for CRPS is often based on studies of outcomes from treatment of other neuropathic pain syndromes.

Physical and occupational therapies

Physical therapy, particularly weight bearing, is one of the keys to recovery of function. Particularly in children, physical therapy combined with behavioral strategies can be highly successful. Development of motor imagery using a mirror box and other techniques has proven to be helpful. Such techniques can be described as 'reprogramming the brain', and aim particularly at the motor cortex changes now known to occur. Physical therapy and, to a lesser extent, occupational therapy can reduce pain and improve active mobility in CRPS I.

The order of physical therapy strategies appears to be important: laterality recognition, followed by imagining movement, followed by mirror movements.

Psychological therapy

Only one prospective randomized study has evaluated cognitive behavioral treatment (CBT) in children and adults with CRPS, showing a long-lasting reduction in all symptoms in both groups. In our own experience CBT, which helps patients develop coping skills for managing stress in CRPS pain, is a crucial component of treatment and is essential in CRPS of long duration.

Pharmacological management

Non-steroidal anti-inflammatory drugs. There are no studies of non-steroidal anti-inflammatory drugs (NSAIDs) in CRPS. However, from clinical experience NSAIDs help in mild to moderate pain.

Opioids. There are no studies of opioids in CRPS. In the presence of severe pain, opioids should be at least partially effective, as they are effective for other neuropathic pain.

Calcitonin is a hormone produced in the thyroid gland. It has a hypocalcemic effect, inhibiting osteoclastic bone resorption and increasing urinary excretion of calcium and phosphorus. Calcitonin also has a central analgesic effect, but the underlying mechanism is unknown. Naturally occurring porcine calcitonin, synthetic salmon calcitonin and synthetic human calcitonin are all in clinical use. Calcitonin is usually administered by intramuscular or subcutaneous injection, but the intranasal route is also frequently used. Randomized controlled trials (RCTs) to evaluate the benefits of calcitonin in patients with CRPS have shown a small effect at best.

Corticosteroids. Two small single-blind RCTs reported a decrease in pain in patients with acute CRPS after treatment with corticosteroids. The limited sample size of these two studies (n = 23 and n = 36), and the fact that the studies were not double blinded must be taken into account when considering the significance of the results.

Bisphosphonates. CRPS is associated with increased bone resorption and patchy osteoporosis. Three double-blind RCTs reported that patients treated with alendronate intravenously (7.5 mg/day for 3 days) or orally (40 mg/day) had less pain, tenderness and swelling, and improved motion compared with those receiving placebo; however, the very small sample sizes (n = 20–32) in these studies preclude any firm conclusion that bisphosphonates are useful therapies.

Tricyclic antidepressants. Although antidepressants are known to be effective in the treatment of neuropathic pain, only one trial has been conducted in patients with CRPS. Of the 48 patients with CRPS type II evaluated, those who took clomipramine exhibited greater pain relief than did those who received acetylsalicylic acid (ASA; aspirin).

Anticonvulsants. Although these are effective treatments for neuropathic pain, their use for the treatment of CRPS has not been evaluated, with the exception of one trial that evaluated gabapentin in 307 people with neuropathic pain, 85 of whom had CRPS types I or II. Those who received gabapentin exhibited greater improvement than did those who received placebo.

Capsaicin. A meta-analysis of therapies for CRPS and peripheral neuropathy demonstrated that topical application of capsaicin (an alkaloid derived from chili peppers) decreased pain intensity. However, it was difficult to blind the study because of the burning sensation associated with capsaicin treatment.

Intravenous lidocaine (lignocaine) is effective in CRPS I and II in terms of reducing spontaneous evoked pain.

Gamma-aminobutyric acid (GABA) agonists. Intrathecal baclofen effectively relieves the dystonia of CRPS.

Modulation of the sympathetic nervous system. The efficacy of phentolamine and of intravenous regional sympathetic block with guanethidine has not been confirmed in RCTs.

Local anesthetic blockade of the sympathetic chain is a standard clinical therapy for CRPS, but the scarcity of RCTs precludes any conclusion concerning the effectiveness of this intervention. A qualitative systematic review of observational studies of this therapy suggests that less than one-third of patients treated by local anesthetic sympathetic blockade obtain full pain relief. This rate of success is acceptable to many patients and clinicians, yet its magnitude could be attributed to placebo response, natural history or regression to the mean. Treatment early in the course of CRPS appears to be more effective than in well-established CRPS.

Invasive procedures

Invasive procedures should not be considered in the early treatment of CRPS. They are invasive, there is a scarcity of evidence to support their use and, to date, only short follow-up periods have been reported. These therapies should, therefore, be offered only in the context of multidisciplinary treatment and after careful screening and patient selection. Nevertheless, the dilemma associated with the use of invasive techniques is that they seem to be more successful when applied early in the course of the condition. Thus, a stepwise approach to non-invasive treatment should be pursued with deliberate speed.

Surgical sympathectomy. Definitive sympathectomy by surgical division, neurolytic nerve blocks or radiofrequency lesioning is not recommended as none provides long-lasting pain relief. In fact, surgical sympathectomy frequently leads to new or worsened chronic pain.

Spinal cord stimulation (SCS). Case series of treatments such as peripheral nerve stimulation with an implantable programmable generator and spinal cord stimulation report up to 15% of the systems have to be removed owing to lack of lasting pain relief. The only RCT to date reported that 37% of a small sample of 36 patients achieved substantial improvement in their global assessment but there was no improvement in functional status assessed 2 years after treatment started. This study did not employ intensive cognitive behavioral therapy to address functional deficits.

Nevertheless, in severe and refractory cases of CRPS a trial of SCS may be reasonable, particularly if any pain relief is paired with behavioral and physical therapies targeted at improving function and potentially reversing neuroplastic and behavioral changes associated with CRPS. Objective evidence of improvement should first be documented in a temporary trial (e.g. abolition of tremor, improved range of movement, ability to bear weight) before proceeding with the implantation of stimulating electrodes. In some patients with very severe CRPS causing complete limitation of movement of a limb, reversal of this situation occurs within a few hours of starting a trial of SCS. The trial can be continued on an outpatient basis.

Epidural clonidine. The same judicious approach as described for SCS should be taken with epidural clonidine. Although some case series have reported beneficial effects, there are no rigorous data for patients with CRPS. However, a trial of epidural clonidine may be appropriate for patients with intractable CRPS, and may help the patient start weight-bearing and other activity focused on functional restoration.

Preventive strategies

Patients known to have had a previous episode of CRPS, or who are currently suffering from CRPS, are at risk of triggering or exacerbating CRPS if they undergo surgery of the affected limb or suffer trauma to the limb. Preventive measures should be initiated as soon as possible. Stellate ganglion block before upper limb surgery in patients with a prior history of CRPS reduced the recurrence rate in one study. In a second study intravenous regional anesthesia with lidocaine (lignocaine) and clonidine was also effective. On theoretical grounds a number of the pharmacotherapeutic options described above may be effective but have not been studied. In our experience, perioperative low-dose ketamine infusion, combined with gabapentin or pregabalin, has proven valuable. Rarely, epidural clonidine is used where there is severe risk of CRPS exacerbation.

Prognosis

The severity of CRPS, rather than its etiology, seems to determine the disease course. Thus, early intervention to reduce the severity of CRPS is vital. In CRPS I, causal fractures have a higher resolution rate (91%) than causal sprain (78%) or other etiology (55%). In CRPS II, more than 60% of patients were unchanged after 1 year of intensive therapy. However, studies of outcome after more than 1 year of treatment with new techniques are now needed.

Key points – complex regional pain syndrome

- Complex regional pain syndrome (CRPS) involves abnormalities in sensation, motor and sympathetic function, as well as edema and abnormal sweating, with possible trophic changes.
- The involvement of the sympathetic nervous system in CRPS is likely, but detailed mechanisms differ among patients and remain unclear.
- Diagnosis requires the presence of a number of symptoms and signs in the areas of sensory, motor and sympathetic function in the absence of any other condition that might account for the symptoms.
- Intravenous regional sympathetic blockade with guanethidine or systemic phentolamine lack efficacy.
- Local anesthetic blockade of the sympathetic chain is a default clinical treatment for acute CRPS, but the scarcity of data from randomized controlled trials precludes any firm conclusion regarding its effectiveness.
- Sympathectomy by surgical division, chemical neurolysis or radiofrequency lesioning should be avoided.
- Pharmacotherapy largely relies on studies of treatment of other types of neuropathic pain.
- Severe CRPS warrants a cognitive behavioral treatment program and may require a trial of spinal cord stimulation.
- New strategies in 'reprogramming the brain' may be able to address the neuroplastic changes that occur with CRPS.

Key references

Baron R, Fields HL, Janig W et al. National Institutes of Health Workshop: reflex sympathetic dystrophy/complex regional pain syndromes – state-of-the-science. *Anesth Analg* 2002;95:1812–16.

Baron R, Janig W. Complex regional pain syndromes—how do we escape the diagnostic trap? *Lancet* 2004;364:1739–41.

Cepeda MS, Carr DB, Lau J. Local anesthetic sympathetic blockade for complex regional pain syndrome. *Cochrane Database Syst Rev* 2005, issue 4. CD004598. www.thecochranelibrary.com.

Compston JE, Rosen CJ. *Fast Facts: Osteoporosis*, 6th edn. Oxford: Health Press Limited, 2009.

Drummond PD. Sensory disturbances in complex regional pain syndrome: clinical observations, autonomic interactions, and possible mechanisms. *Pain Med* 2010;11: 1257–66.

Harden N, Bruehl S, Stanton-Hicks M, Wilson PR. Proposed new diagnostic criteria for complex regional pain syndrome. *Pain Med* 2007;8:326–31.

Maihofner C, Baron R, DeCol R et al. The motor system shows adaptive changes in complex regional pain syndrome. *Brain* 2007;130:2671–87.

Moseley GL. Graded motor imagery is effective for long-standing complex regional pain syndrome: a randomised controlled trial. *Pain* 2004;108:192–8.

Perez RS, Kwakkel G, Zuurmond WW, de Lange JJ. Treatment of reflex sympathetic dystrophy (CRPS type 1): a research synthesis of 21 randomized clinical trials. *J Pain Symptom Manage* 2001;21:511–26.

Veldman PH, Reynen HM, Arntz IE, Goris RJ. Signs and symptoms of reflex sympathetic dystrophy: prospective study of 829 patients. *Lancet* 1993;342:1012–16.

Walker SM, Cousins MJ. Complex regional pain syndromes: including "reflex sympathetic dystrophy" and "causalgia". *Anaesth Intensive Care* 1997;25:113–25.

Diabetic neuropathy

Diabetic neuropathy (DN) refers to a group of heterogeneous disorders that affect the autonomic and peripheral nervous systems of approximately 20% of patients with diabetes mellitus. The neuropathy may or may not be painful, though over 45% of individuals who have had diabetes for 25 years will experience painful DN.

Patients report a spectrum of symptoms ranging from mildly disturbing tingling to severe pain that can interfere with sleep and normal activities. Pain may be burning and constant and there may be intermittent electric-shock-like symptoms. Allodynia may be present as well as dysesthesias. The degree of nerve damage does not correlate with pain intensity, and patients can develop insensitive feet without preceding pain or paresthesias. Table 5.1 lists the major types of painful diabetic neuropathy. Small-fiber neuropathy results in loss of ability to feel pressure on the skin of the feet leading to the development of pressure sores, which commonly become infected and painful. All of the other types of neuropathy can be painful.

Pathophysiology. Persistent hyperglycemia is the primary factor responsible for nerve damage. Hyperglycemia increases oxidative stress in nerve cells because of an excess of polyol (sugar alcohol) in the aldose reductase pathway and increases production of diacylglycerol, which subsequently activates protein kinase C.

In 11% of diabetic patients, neurological signs are evident before the diagnosis of diabetes, which suggests that the pathogenic mechanism in some patients is only loosely linked to hyperglycemia.

Glycemia-independent theories include autoimmune damage, damage due to hypoxia, and decreased synthesis of nerve-growth factor and neurotrophins.

Damage to peripheral neurons results in spontaneous firing and increased sensitivity of nociceptors (see Chapter 1). Increased input to

TABLE 5.1

Types of painful diabetic neuropathy

Type	Description/symptoms
Acute mononeuropathy	• Normal tendon reflexes • Vascular obstruction • Truncal neuropathy
Autonomic neuropathy	• Silent myocardial infarction • Gastroparesis • Bladder dysfunction • Disturbed neurovascular flow
Compressive neuropathy	• Sensory loss in nerve distribution (e.g. carpal tunnel syndrome)
Large fiber neuropathy	• Motor weakness • Impaired vibration perception
Small fiber neuropathy	• Paresthesias • No motor deficit • Defective heat sensation • Later, progressive hypoalgesia • Risk of foot ulceration
Proximal motor neuropathy	• Pain in thighs • Weakness • Diminished tendon reflexes • Diabetic amyotrophy

the spinal dorsal horn results in central sensitization and increased firing of dorsal horn neurons. The spontaneous firing of peripheral neurons is associated with a change in the distribution of voltage-gated sodium channels, with an altered subtype representation (e.g. of $Na_V1.8$). This offers a future potential for precisely targeted treatment (e.g. $Na_V1.8$ blockers) at the periphery.

Diagnosis of DN rests heavily on a careful medical history. The American Academy of Neurology recommends that patients with diabetes and neuropathy should provide a medical history and undergo a neurological examination, as well as a nerve-conduction-velocity study, quantitative sensory testing and quantitative autonomic function testing. The last two tests evaluate the patient's reaction to vibration, light touch, pain and changes in temperature, as well as proprioception and autonomic function. However, these laboratory tests are not necessary to make the diagnosis of DN and to begin treatment of pain.

To allow primary care providers to detect neuropathy in people with diabetes in clinical practice easily, a simple diagnostic tool has been developed and validated – the diabetic neuropathy symptom score.

Primary care providers should ask patients about unsteadiness in walking and the presence of pain, paresthesia or numbness. Each symptom adds one point for a maximum possible score of 4. A score of 1 or higher is considered diagnostic for polyneuropathy.

During the physical examination, clinicians can simply, rapidly and reliably screen patients for polyneuropathy using the vibration test. This test comprises the application of a 128-Hz tuning fork to the bony prominence bilaterally situated at the dorsum of the toe just proximal to the nail bed. The patient is then asked to report the perception of both the onset and the subsiding of the sensation of vibration. Testing should be conducted twice on each toe. Peripheral neuropathy is diagnosed if more than half of the responses are incorrect (five incorrect responses or more out of ten tests).

Prevention. Complications of diabetes mellitus (including infections) are more common with poor glycemic control. Randomized controlled trials (RCTs) have shown that maintenance of near-normal blood glucose levels with intensive insulin treatment is the best approach to primary and secondary prevention of late diabetic complications such as diabetic neuropathy, the prevalence of which may be reduced by 64%.

Metabolic treatment seems to be a promising approach. Aldose reductase inhibitors suppress the accumulation of alcohol sugars in nerve cells and thus improve conduction velocity; however, the clinical importance of these surrogates is inconclusive.

Pharmacological management. Tricyclic antidepressants (TCAs) and anticonvulsants are the medications of choice for neuropathic pain, but side effects are common.

The National Institute for Health and Clinical Excellence (England and Wales) recommends a stepwise approach.
- Step 1: paracetamol (acetaminophen) or ASA (aspirin).
- Step 2: TCAs (see below) with appropriate medical cautions, particularly in the elderly.
- Step 3: gabapentin.
- Opioids are reserved for pain clinics.

In the USA, the Mayo Foundation recommends duloxetine, slow-release oxycodone, pregabalin or a TCA as a first-line treatment as these are all supported by findings from more than two RCTs. The only two drugs specifically licensed for DN are duloxetine and pregabalin.

Antidepressants. The analgesic benefit of TCAs can be explained by several pharmacological mechanisms: they inhibit the presynaptic uptake of norepinephrine (noradrenaline) and serotonin within nociceptive monoamine pathways and thereby augment analgesia; they interact with opioid receptors; and they block sodium channels, which may account for their analgesic effect in topical creams.

The effectiveness of TCAs for DN has been confirmed in meta-analyses of RCTs. Trial findings have indicated that 1 in 4 individuals given a TCA experiences substantial pain relief (at least 50% relief). However, 1 in 3 individuals develops minor side effects and 1 in 17 stops the medication because of the severity of side effects. The best-studied TCAs are amitriptyline (25–150 mg/day), imipramine and desipramine (desipramine is not licensed in the UK).

Newer antidepressants such as selective serotonin-reuptake inhibitors (SSRIs) are preferable to TCAs for the treatment of depression, but SSRIs do not inhibit the reuptake of both serotonin and norepinephrine, which appears to be necessary for effect against DN. Emerging data on the treatment of neuropathic pain with the 'balanced' serotonin–norepinephrine-reuptake inhibitor (SNRI) duloxetine are promising and this drug is now approved for DN in some countries. An older antidepressant with similar SNRI properties, venlafaxine, is also used to treat peripheral DN.

The main side effects of TCAs are dry mouth and sedation, both of which are the result of the antimuscarinic activity of the drugs. Low starting doses and careful titration may help to minimize these effects. Orthostatic hypotension, tachycardia, urinary retention and constipation, sometimes associated with TCAs, may also pose a problem in the elderly. Because disturbances of cardiac rhythm may be potentiated by TCAs, a baseline electrocardiogram should be taken before therapy is started, particularly in the elderly. The main side effects of SNRI antidepressants are nausea and vomiting; venlafaxine is associated with an increase in blood pressure at the higher doses needed for analgesia.

Treatment of patients with neuropathic pain and cardiovascular disease should begin with anticonvulsants or antidepressants with SNRI properties such as duloxetine or venlafaxine, given the increased risk of cardiovascular events associated with the use of TCAs.

Anticonvulsants. Many anticonvulsants block voltage-dependent sodium channels and suppress peripherally generated ectopic impulse activity. However, some anticonvulsants such as gabapentin and pregabalin exert their effect through non-sodium-channel mechanisms. They act upon a modulatory site of neuronal calcium channels. Gabanoid binding at this site reduces calcium influx at nerve terminals and reduces the release of excitatory neurotransmitters.

The effectiveness of anticonvulsants has been confirmed in meta-analyses of RCTs. As with antidepressants, 1 in 3 individuals given anticonvulsants experiences pain relief. However, 1 in 4 individuals experiences minor adverse effects or severe symptoms that cause them to stop taking the medication.

Carbamazepine, 400–1000 mg/day, is traditionally used for neuropathic pain. The more recently introduced anticonvulsant gabapentin, 1800–3600 mg/day, is also widely used for neuropathic pain; evidence from RCTs suggests that it is not superior to carbamazepine in terms of effectiveness or common side effects. However, side effects can be more severe with carbamazepine. It is not clear if pregabalin is superior to gabapentin, but pregabalin does not require lengthy titration. Trial data show that 1 in 5 individuals given pregabalin, 150–600 mg/day, experiences pain relief.

Infrequent cases of Stevens–Johnson syndrome and lymphoid hyperplasia have been reported in patients treated with carbamazepine, but not in those treated with gabapentin or pregabalin.

One in ten individuals taking gabapentin or pregabalin stops taking the medication because of severe adverse events such as dizziness, somnolence or ataxia. The adverse events are dose related: trial data have shown that, with daily doses of 150 mg, only 1 in 39 individuals taking pregabalin discontinues the medication because of adverse events. Perhaps because the clinical picture indicates fewer severe adverse events with gabapentin and pregabalin, clinicians have widely adopted these gabanoids as first-line agents for the treatment of neuropathic pain. Pregabalin is now approved specifically for DN in a number of countries.

Opioids are increasingly used for the treatment of refractory pain, regardless of etiology. The efficacy of opioids in neuropathic pain is established in RCTs, but their long-term effectiveness and side effects have not been well defined and abuse of prescription drugs is a growing problem. Troublesome side effects, such as nausea and vomiting and sedation, are common. Moreover, adverse effects from longer-term exposure, such as hypogonadism, are now documented. Methadone must be used cautiously with slow titration because of its biphasic hepatic metabolism that may be affected by co-medications, such as antidepressants and anticonvulsants, frequently co-prescribed for pain.

A meta-analysis of RCTs has shown that tramadol, an analgesic with a dual mechanism of action (i.e. activating both opioid receptors and descending inhibitory pain systems) reduces pain intensity in patients with postherpetic neuralgia and DN at mean doses of 210 mg/day. As with studies that have evaluated traditional opioids, the follow-up periods in the tramadol studies were short. No conclusion can therefore be made as to whether tolerance causes a decline in effectiveness with chronic use, as might be expected for that portion of the drug's effect that is opioid related.

Systematic reviews of RCTs have revealed that about 80% of patients receiving opioids experience at least one adverse event. The small number of patients in these trials, and the short duration of follow-up, mean that key concerns regarding tolerance and addiction risk have not yet been answered.

Opioid receptors are coupled to ion channels via G proteins. When activated, these receptors modulate calcium and potassium entry into the neuronal membrane. Opioids decrease nociceptive transmission and produce analgesia by hyperpolarizing nociceptive cell membranes, shortening the duration of their action potentials and inhibiting the release of excitatory mediators. However, opioids can also induce a state of increased pain sensitivity (hyperalgesia), even after a relatively short period of exposure. Explanations for this paradoxical effect include prolongation of the neuronal action potential, activation of descending facilitatory pathways, activation of glial cell facilitatory mechanisms, modulation of N-methyl D-aspartate receptors and increased release of dynorphin in the spinal cord. Opioid-induced hyperalgesia may limit the long-term effectiveness of these drugs in some patients with chronic pain.

Postherpetic neuralgia

Postherpetic neuralgia (PHN) is pain that persists after the vesicular rash of acute herpes zoster (shingles) has resolved. Rarely, the condition occurs despite the absence of an obvious rash. The associated pain is usually mild or moderate in intensity, but it may be excruciating. Typically, a single dermatome is involved, but occasionally more than one is affected. Acute herpes zoster is common, developing in up to 20% of people, though PHN is predominantly a disease of older people (see below).

Pathophysiology. Acute herpes zoster results from reactivation of varicella zoster virus (VZV) that has remained latent in neurons of the spinal dorsal root ganglia since an earlier infection, usually childhood chickenpox (in more than 90% of cases). Risk factors for virus activation are older age, malignant disease including lymphoma, and immunosuppression due to drugs or disease.

When reactivated, the virus replicates and spreads outwards to sensory ganglia and afferent peripheral nerves. The virus causes neuronal loss and inflammatory infiltrates in the dorsal root ganglia, nerves and nerve roots. These changes trigger the pathophysiology associated with neuropathic pain (see Chapter 1, pages 14–18). Interestingly, animal studies have suggested that even in the latent phase the presence of the virus may induce abnormalities in afferent nerve function.

Natural history. Advancing age is an important risk factor for developing PHN. After acute herpes zoster infection, 2% of patients under 60 years old develop PHN, but this figure progressively increases to about 50% with advancing age. The apparent severity of PHN reported in RCTs is higher, perhaps reflecting a referral bias. Other risk factors are the severity of the acute zoster lesions and the intensity of the acute pain.

The duration of PHN is highly variable: at least 30% of all individuals with this type of pain will continue to have severe pain 1 year after the onset of herpes zoster.

Diagnosis. PHN is diagnosed on the basis of a history of shingles and the presence of persistent neuropathic pain in the affected dermatome. Symptoms are experienced around the area of skin where the shingles outbreak first occurred. Patients describe a sharp jabbing burning pain or a deep aching pain, with extreme sensitivity to touch and temperature change. They sometimes describe an itching sensation or numbness and, in instances of cranial nerve involvement, their complaint may be considered simply as a headache. PHN often has three distinct types of pain (Table 5.2). Allodynia may result in extreme difficulty wearing clothes and carrying out self-care.

Prevention of PHN is a key strategy as, once developed, PHN is very difficult to treat.

Pediatric VZV vaccination. Prevention starts with pediatric vaccination with VZV, usually around 18 months and then at 10–13 years to prevent infection (ages for vaccination may differ between countries). A range of different pediatric VZV vaccines have been available since 1999, and are funded by governments in some

TABLE 5.2

Types of pain in postherpetic neuralgia

Constant background pain

- Fluctuates in intensity, often burning
- During recovery becomes absent for longer periods before diminishing in intensity

Paroxysmal pain

- Shooting pain through the area

Allodynia (painful hypersensitivity)

- Pain produced by light touch, particularly moving contact with skin
- Present in 90% of patients with postherpetic neuralgia
- Often very distressing
- Frequently last pain type to disappear, if at all

countries. However, the waning of immunity before adulthood has raised questions about the value of pediatric vaccination.

Adult VZV vaccination can be carried out in the 'at-risk' adult over 60 years to prevent VZV reactivation. A large randomized double-blind placebo-controlled trial (n = 35 546 adults > 60 years) investigated vaccination with live attenuated VZV vaccine. The outcome was a reduction in the incidence of herpes zoster (59 vaccinations to prevent one case) and PHN (802 vaccinations to prevent one case). In immunocompromised recipients of bone marrow transplants, vaccination with an inactive VZV vaccine also reduces incidence of PHN.

Antiviral treatment. If acute herpes zoster occurs, antiviral treatment should be given as soon as possible to reduce the severity and duration of the acute zoster episode and thus indirectly decrease risk of PHN (there is no direct effect of antiviral treatment on PHN). Meta-analyses of RCTs have indicated that aciclovir (acyclovir) reduces the severity and duration of herpes zoster and acute zoster-associated pain. Aciclovir should be given at 800 mg five times daily for 7 days. However, as the condition is often well established before treatment is started, antiviral therapy may be of limited effectiveness.

Effective pain treatment in the acute phase reduces risk of PHN. A 90-day course of amitriptyline, started during the acute herpes zoster attack, was found in an RCT to reduce pain intensity assessed 6 months later.

Pharmacological management of established PHN. Overall, pharmacological treatment of PHN tends to be unsatisfactory. It is not clear why some patients obtain good pain relief while others do not. It may reflect: different underlying mechanisms among patients despite similar initiating events; genetically determined variation in pain response (see Chapter 1) or differing influences of psychological and environmental factors.

Sympathetic blockade. Anecdotal observations of prompt pain reduction and apparent truncation of the evolution of acute shingles into PHN have led to the use of sympathetic blockade during the acute phase of this viral illness. However, supportive evidence from RCTs is lacking.

Systemic corticosteroids. Meta-analyses of RCTs show that corticosteroids do not prevent PHN.

Tricyclic antidepressants are useful for PHN, as in DN (see pages 62–3). SSRIs do not seem to be effective.

Anticonvulsants can effectively relieve postherpetic pain, as shown by meta-analyses of RCTs. The degree of effect is similar to that reported for DN (see pages 63–4). Gabapentin, pregabalin and sodium valproate have been reported to be effective in PHN. In a comparative study of gabapentin versus nortriptyline, pain relief results were similar, but gabapentin was better tolerated.

Capsaicin relieves pain associated with PHN. Capsaicin binds to vanilloid receptors on C and Aδ fibers, and provokes pain at initial application because of the release of substance P from the peripheral nerve terminals. This thermal cue makes blinding in RCTs difficult and may positively bias the benefits observed in such trials. Pain relief on repeated application of capsaicin reflects depletion of excitatory mediators from peripheral nerve endings.

Key points – diabetic and postherpetic neuropathic pain

- Persistent hyperglycemia is the primary factor responsible for nerve damage in diabetes mellitus.
- Maintenance of near-normal blood glucose levels is the best approach to primary and secondary prevention of diabetic neuropathy (DN).
- DN affects the autonomic and peripheral nervous systems.
- Tricyclic antidepressants, serotonin–norepinephrine-reuptake inhibitor (SNRI) antidepressants and anticonvulsants are the medications of choice for neuropathic pain, but side effects are common. Pregabalin has emerged as a specifically approved drug for DN. Duloxetine has also gained approval as a specific indication for DN in some countries.
- The use of opioids for the treatment of neuropathic pain remains controversial because the literature has not established the long-term safety and efficacy of these drugs.
- Postherpetic neuralgia (PHN) is pain that persists after the vesicular rash of herpes zoster has resolved.
- During an attack of acute herpes zoster (shingles), reactivation of the varicella zoster virus, previously dormant in the dorsal root ganglia, induces inflammation and neuronal destruction.
- Tricyclic antidepressants and anticonvulsants are useful therapies.
- Physical, psychological and social consequences of PHN should all receive attention.
- Once developed PHN is difficult to manage and thus efforts to prevent PHN are crucial via: prevention of varicella zoster virus (VZV) infection, boosting VZV immunity or treating at the time of acute herpes zoster infection, including effective treatment of the acute pain.

Opioids. Discussion on the use of opioids in DN (see pages 64–5) applies equally to use in PHN or other neuropathic chronic pain.

Lidocaine skin patch. A meta-analysis of RCTs of topical lidocaine (lignocaine) patches for PHN reached no firm conclusion regarding effect.

Invasive approaches may need to be considered for severe neuropathic pain that does not respond to the usual treatments. Systemic lidocaine infusion may be used to bring a severe exacerbation of pain under control. Systemic ketamine infusion may be required in extreme situations.

In rare cases, a trial of spinal cord stimulation (SCS) may be warranted prior to considering permanent implantation of an SCS system – particularly in patients who are intolerant of drugs.

Non-pharmacological management. Trials to evaluate the effectiveness of transcutaneous electrical nerve stimulation (TENS) for chronic pain have been inconclusive owing to the small number of participants, a lack of placebo control, a lack of long-term assessment and inadequate details of the stimulation variables most likely to provide pain relief.

Treatment of psychosocial sequelae of PHN may improve a patient's ability to lead a normal life. Psychological techniques such as 'desensitization' (a strategy to reduce the response to neuropathic pain) may be invaluable.

Key references

Anon. Intensive blood-glucose control with sulphonylureas or insulin compared with conventional treatment and risk of complications in patients with type 2 diabetes (UKPDS 33). UK Prospective Diabetes Study (UKPDS) Group. *Lancet* 1998;352:837–53.

Boulton AJ, Vinik AI, Arezzo JC et al. Diabetic neuropathies: a statement by the American Diabetes Association. *Diabetes Care* 2005;28:956–62.

Cepeda MS, Farrar JT. Economic evaluation of oral treatments for neuropathic pain. *J Pain* 2006;7:119–28.

Chandra K, Shafiq N, Pandhi P et al. Gabapentin versus nortriptyline in post-herpetic neuralgia patients: a randomized, double-blind clinical trial—the GONIP Trial. *Int J Clin Pharmacol Ther* 2006;44:358–63.

Collins SL, Moore RA, McQuay H, Wiffen P. Antidepressants and anticonvulsants for diabetic neuropathy and postherpetic neuralgia: a quantitative systematic review. *J Pain Symptom Manage* 2000;20:449–58.

Eisenberg E, McNicol ED, Carr DB. Efficacy and safety of opioid agonists in the treatment of neuropathic pain of nonmalignant origin: systematic review and meta-analysis of randomized controlled trials. *JAMA* 2005;293:3043–52.

Gajraj NM. Pregabalin: its pharmacology and use in pain management. *Anesth Analg* 2007;105:1805–15.

Greene DA, Stevens MJ, Obrosova I, Feldman EL. Glucose-induced oxidative stress and programmed cell death in diabetic neuropathy. *Eur J Pharmacol* 1999;375:217–23.

Helgason S, Petursson G, Gudmundsson S, Sigurdsson JA. Prevalence of postherpetic neuralgia after a first episode of herpes zoster: prospective study with long term follow up. *BMJ* 2000;321:794–6.

Jung BF, Johnson RW, Griffin DR, Dworkin RH. Risk factors for postherpetic neuralgia in patients with herpes zoster. *Neurology* 2004;62:1545–51.

Kalso E, Edwards JE, Moore RA, McQuay HJ. Opioids in chronic non-cancer pain: systematic review of efficacy and safety. *Pain* 2004;112:372–80.

Kimberlin DW, Whitley RJ. Varicella-zoster vaccine for the prevention of herpes zoster. *N Engl J Med* 2007;356:1338–43.

Oxman MN, Levin MJ, Johnson GR et al. A vaccine to prevent herpes zoster and postherpetic neuralgia in older adults. *N Engl J Med* 2005;352:2271–84.

Santee JA. Corticosteroids for herpes zoster: what do they accomplish? *Am J Clin Dermatol* 2002;3:517–24.

Scobie IN, Samaras K. *Fast Facts: Diabetes Mellitus*, 3rd edn. Oxford: Health Press Limited, 2009.

Tolle T, Freynhagen R, Versavel M et al. Pregabalin for relief of neuropathic pain associated with diabetic neuropathy: a randomized, double–blind study. *Eur J Pain* 2008;12:203–13.

Wiffen P, Collins S, McQuay H et al. Anticonvulsant drugs for acute and chronic pain. *Cochrane Database Syst Rev* 2005, issue 3. CD001133. www.thecochranelibrary.com.

Woo EJ, Ball R, Braun MM. Varicella-zoster vaccine. *N Engl J Med* 2007;357:88.

Wood MJ, Kay R, Dworkin RH et al. Oral acyclovir therapy accelerates pain resolution in patients with herpes zoster: a meta-analysis of placebo-controlled trials. *Clin Infect Dis* 1996;22:341–7.

Central pain is defined by the International Association for the Study of Pain (IASP) as 'pain initiated or caused by a primary lesion (or dysfunction) of the central nervous system (CNS)'. It has been suggested that 'or dysfunction' be deleted as peripheral nerve lesions can eventually lead to dysfunction in the CNS.

Spinal cord injury (SCI; trauma or disease) (Figure 6.1) and stroke are the most common causes of lesions in the spinal cord or brain and brainstem that cause central pain, but there are many others (Table 6.1). It has now been recognized that epilepsy can be painful as can Parkinson's disease. Multiple sclerosis causes central pain in about 60% of patients.

Pathophysiology

Post-stroke pain. Conditions sufficient for the generation of central pain were previously thought to be an imbalance between spinothalamic

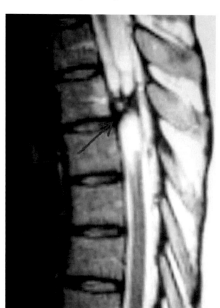

Figure 6.1 MRI scan showing spinal cord transection at the thoracic level secondary to trauma (see arrow). The patient suffered from paraplegia and spontaneous pain and allodynia in both legs.

TABLE 6.1

Sources of central pain

- Vascular lesions in the brain and spinal cord
- Infarction
- Hemorrhage
- Vascular malformation
- Multiple sclerosis
- Traumatic spinal cord injury
- Cordotomy
- Traumatic brain injury

- Syringomyelia and syringobulbia
- Tumors
- Abscesses
- Inflammatory diseases other than multiple sclerosis
- Myelitis caused by viruses or syphilis
- Epilepsy
- Parkinson's disease

From Wasner G, Baron R. Central pain syndromes. In: Castro-Lopes J, Raja S, Schmelz M, eds. *Pain 2008 – An Updated Review. IASP Refresher Course Syllabus.* Seattle: IASP Press, 2008.

system (caused by a lesion in that system) and medial lemniscal pathways. This is now known to be untrue. However, Craig et al. have provided evidence of a key role of ventromedial posterior thalamic lesions that allow disinhibition of a medial spinothalamic tract projecting via the medial dorsal nucleus of the thalamus to the anterior cingulated cortex (limbic system) – this appears to be associated with the burning nature of central post-stroke pain and also generates cold hypoesthesia. In 2007, Kim et al. reported that lesions limited to the ventral caudal thalamic nucleus may produce a similar presentation of central post-stroke pain. Thus, there are several sites of lesion associated with post-stroke pain; unfortunately, this does not yet provide insight into the precise mechanisms of such pain (see Henry 2007).

Pain following SCI. The study of central pain arising from SCI has been more productive than that of post-stroke pain. Key insight was provided from a 5-year follow-up study of SCI pain by Siddall et al., which reported that at-level SCI pain often progressed to below-level pain – suggesting spinal and supraspinal mechanisms triggered by at-level SCI pain predispose to below-level 'central' pain.

A number of putative mechanisms have emerged from basic, clinical, epidemiological and brain-imaging research:

- loss of balance between different sensory channels
- loss of spinal inhibitory mechanisms
- presence of pattern generators above the level of SCI in the spinal cord or supraspinal relay nuclei
- synaptic plasticity changes
- spinal and supraspinal microglial activation (see Figure 1.8).

Recent brain-imaging studies report neuroplastic changes in the brain that correlate with severity of post-SCI pain (see Figure 1.10).

Overall, complex processes appear to operate at the level of a 'spinal generator' and a 'supraspinal generator/amplifier'. The relative roles of each level in at-level and below-level SCI pain remain to be clarified. An important aspect is the relationship of post-SCI neuropathic pain and hyperreflexic responses (autonomic hyperreflexia). It has long been known that complete SCI lesions remove descending inhibitory control and allow severe autonomic mass reflexes. An example is severe vasoconstriction in response to a noxious stimulus – the vasoconstriction increases blood pressure which, in turn, activates vasomotor and other brainstem and brain structures, resulting in exacerbation of neuropathic pain (Figure 6.2).

Figure 6.2 Spinal cord injury, autonomic dysreflexia and pain. After a complete T4–6 transection, noxious stimulation below the lesion, such as a severely distended or infected bladder, results in a barrage of input to the spinal cord. (1) In the absence of any descending inhibitory processes an exaggerated sympathetic reflex response occurs, with vasoconstriction of gut vasculature; increased blood pressure activates barroreceptors and the brainstem vasomotor center, impinging on the periaqueductal gray (PAG) area that is a watershed for respiratory and hemodynamic control. Neuropathic pain perception increases as a result of these central changes. Also, vagal nerve activation results in compensatory bradycardia, nasal congestion, profuse sweating and flushing in the face and neck – as well as a pounding headache. (2) Noxious input to the cord also results in reflex activation of muscle without any normal inhibitory control (upper motor neuron lesion). Thus, spastic responses occur, which may be painful.

Diagnosis

Lesions in the brain. Stroke is the most common cause of neuropathic pain related to brain lesions. More than 8% of all stroke patients suffer with central pain. In view of the high incidence of stroke, about 90% of all central pain is associated with stroke. Because stroke is associated with communication difficulties, the high prevalence of central pain was not recognized until quite recently. Previously it was erroneously believed that only thalamic lesions resulted in central pain. Now the diagnosis of 'thalamic syndrome' is reserved for

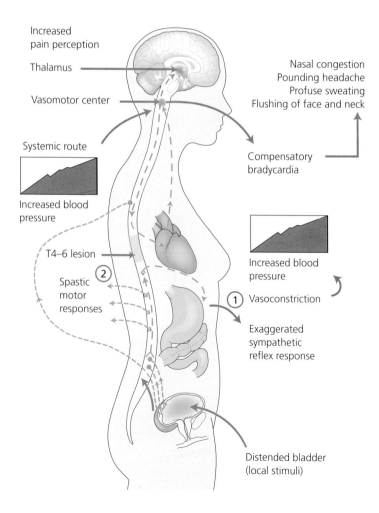

thalamic lesions and otherwise the diagnosis of 'post-stroke pain' is used.

Post-stroke pain is usually located within the area of loss of sensation caused by the stroke, though sometimes only part of the area is affected. CRPS of the paretic arm may occur (see Chapter 4), but this is rare. Importantly, it has been suggested that some pain syndromes associated with stroke are initiated at the periphery: for example, nociceptive pain in shoulder–arm due to subluxation of the scapulohumeral joint, neuropathic pain related to spasticity, and diabetic neuropathy reflecting the significant co-incidence of stroke and diabetes.

Spinal cord injury. Unfortunately, traumatic SCI is common, particularly in young men. In Europe it is estimated that there are currently 300 000 people with SCI and there are about 11 000 new cases per year. In a 5-year follow-up study in Australia, Siddall et al. reported that 34% had below-level neuropathic pain which was deemed to be central pain (Table 6.2). A further 41% had at-level neuropathic pain that probably started at the peripheral level, but usually became 'centralized'. Musculoskeletal and visceral pain contributed to an overall prevalence of 81% of participants reporting pain. There was a strong correlation between the presence of both types of neuropathic pain at 5 years and at earlier time points, pointing to the need to start treating the pain early to prevent the maladaptive changes described in Chapter 1, rather than 'waiting for the pain to go away'.

An IASP taxonomy of post-SCI pain types has been promulgated (see Table 6.2), based on an earlier proposal by Siddall et al. in 1997. This has facilitated comparison of studies using the same terminology. It is important to differentiate non-neuropathic pain, which is present in 60% of SCI patients at 5 years, and which includes: mechanical spinal instability; painful muscle spasms; and secondary overuse syndromes (e.g. of the shoulder joint in paraplegics). Visceral pain may be associated with nociceptive visceral pathology, though in many cases no pathology is found and the pain is presumed to be below-level neuropathic pain (e.g. bladder and rectal pain).

TABLE 6.2

IASP taxonomy of pain following spinal cord injury

Broad type (tier one)	Broad system (tier two)	Specific structures and pathology (tier three)
Nociceptive	Musculoskeletal	Bone, joint, muscle trauma or inflammation
		Mechanical instability
		Muscle spasm
		Secondary or overuse syndrome
	Visceral	For example, renal calculus, bowel dysfunction, sphincter dysfunction
		Dysreflexic headache
Neuropathic	Above level	Compressive mononeuropathies
		Complex regional pain syndromes
	At level	Nerve root compression (including cauda equina)
		Syringomyelia
		Spinal cord trauma/ischemia (e.g. transitional zone)
		Dual-level cord and root trauma (double lesion syndrome)
	Below level	Spinal cord trauma/ischemia (e.g. central dysesthesia syndrome)

From Wasner G, Baron R. Central pain syndromes. In: Castro-Lopes J, Raja S, Schmelz M, eds. *Pain 2008 – An Updated Review. IASP Refresher Course Syllabus.* Seattle: IASP Press, 2008. IASP, International Association for the Study of Pain.

Onset of central pain

Time of pain onset after the initial lesion is extremely variable. In one study of SCI from trauma, 12% of patients had below-level neuropathic pain by 2 weeks after injury, and this had risen to 20%

by 6 months. However, the mean onset time (± implied standard deviation) was 1.8 ± 1.7 years (note the large variance). With stroke, 63% reported onset of central pain within 1 month, 19% between 1 and 6 months and another 19% between 6 and 12 months. Sometimes onset of central pain occurs several years after injury.

Pain sites

Central pain is usually localized in an area of complete or partial loss of sensation, or in an area of abnormal sensation. In SCI, pain may be on both sides of the body below the level of spinal lesion. Sometimes all of the area below the level of the spinal lesion is painful, but in some patients the area may be smaller or even very localized (e.g. bladder or rectum).

Pain character

Usually the neuropathic pain consists of sensations of continuous burning, aching and pricking. Spontaneous or evoked episodes of shooting or stabbing pain also often occur. Patients report that pain can be triggered by emotional situations and may be decreased by intense concentration on work or other mental activities. More than 70% of post-stroke patients suffer allodynia. Allodynia was found to be more common in incomplete SCI (compared with complete SCI) in the 2003 Siddall study.

There is no single pathognomonic description of central pain, though neuropathic descriptors can usually be elicited (see Chapter 2).

Treatment

Central pain is one of the most challenging of all chronic pain conditions. Except for a few exceptions, the underlying condition cannot be successfully treated. However, differential diagnosis of the type of pain is crucial to distinguish nociceptive pain and peripheral neuropathic pain from central pain (see Table 6.2).

The impact of central pain on the individual is usually severe, so a multidisciplinary assessment in a biopsychosocial framework is essential. In many cases a multimodal approach to treatment needs to incorporate pharmacological, psychological and physical therapy strategies. Invasive procedures may be needed in extreme cases.

Psychological, physical and other treatments. Physical therapy has a wide range of roles in patients with post-stroke and SCI pain because of complications related to immobility, postural changes and/or overuse syndromes, or to help relieve symptoms related to neurological disease, such as multiple sclerosis. Mirror visual feedback with 'virtual walking' was effective in 4 patients, but in another study imaginary ankle movement increased neuropathic pain in SCI patients. Further research into such techniques is needed.

The use of cognitive behavioral therapy (CBT) has been evaluated in only one controlled study. At 12-month follow-up, CBT patients had decreased levels of depression and anxiety but no change in pain. Control patients showed no changes.

Pharmacotherapy

Anticonvulsants. In 2008, Finnerup evaluated published randomized controlled trials in central pain with at least 10 participants. An anticonvulsant demonstrating efficacy in central pain in more than one study was pregabalin; those lacking evidence of efficacy were lamotrigine, sodium valproate and carbamazepine.

Antidepressants. A reduction in central post-stroke pain has been reported for amitriptyline, with an NNT of 1.7 (range 1–3) and pain-relieving effects noted from the second week of treatment onwards. Dosage of amitriptyline was increased from 12.5 mg twice daily up to 75 mg daily during the first week and then maintained at this level.

In contrast, in post-SCI central pain, evidence is lacking for efficacy of amitriptyline at doses of 50–125 mg. However, in a study of amitriptyline, 150 mg, in SCI pain there was evidence of analgesic effects, though the high dose raised concerns about potential cardiac toxicity (see Finnerup 2008).

Systemically administered local anesthetics. Some studies of intravenous lidocaine (lignocaine) infusion report short-term efficacy for SCI pain or post-stroke pain. One study supports its use for SCI pain. A study of the oral analog of lidocaine, mexiletine, reported efficacy for SCI pain.

Intravenous anesthetics. A study of the γ-aminobutyric acid (GABA) agonist propofol, given intravenously, reported efficacy, though sedative effects complicated evaluation.

Intravenous ketamine has been reported to reduce continuous or evoked pain in small studies. However, Hocking and Cousins reported no evidence of long-term efficacy in any chronic pain condition when given by the oral route.

Cannabinoids. One study of the cannabinoid tetrahydrocannabinol (THC) at a dose of 10 mg reported efficacy in patients with multiple sclerosis. A second study reported an oromucosal spray based on whole-plant cannabis to be effective in relieving central pain.

Opioids. There is some evidence of short-term efficacy of opioids, but the long-term data that are available are not encouraging, with few patients persisting with opioid therapy.

Invasive procedures

Spinal cord stimulation has proven to be unsuccessful in the large majority of individuals with central pain. The only possible application lies in patients with Brown–Séquard syndrome (unilateral SCI) and pain in a limb with at least partially preserved sensation, which is rare.

Deep brain stimulation has not shown long-term efficacy. Motor cortex stimulation offers more encouraging results, but is still experimental.

Dorsal root entry zone (DREZ) lesioning involves a laminectomy to allow multiple radiofrequency lesions to be made in spinal cord dorsal horn substantia gelatinosa. This technique can provide complete pain relief for many years in patients with avulsion of the roots of the brachial plexus from the spinal cord. Strictly speaking this is a 'peripheral lesion'; however, often there is extensive damage to the spinal cord and the pain is similar to central pain. Patients of this type in whom pharmacotherapy fails should be considered for DREZ lesioning. To reduce the risk of serious complications, including paraplegia and/or extension of the neurological deficit into the neck region, DREZ lesioning should be performed by a neurosurgeon with special training and experience.

Intrathecal drug administration. In SCI pain, one controlled study reported efficacy of morphine plus clonidine given intrathecally, but not for either drug alone. Even with the combination, only 50% of patients responded. Intrathecal baclofen relieves the muscle spasm and associated spasticity in SCI patients and may relieve pain associated with spasticity.

Key points – central pain

- Central pain results from lesions in the brain and brainstem or spinal cord. The most common causes are stroke and traumatic spinal cord injury (SCI), though there are many other causes.
- More than 8% of stroke patients develop central pain. This is probably an underestimate because communication problems may impede diagnosis of pain.
- Onset of post-stroke pain is reported: within 1 month in 63% of patients; between 1 and 6 months in 19%; and in a further 19% between 6 and 12 months. Sometimes onset occurs several years after the injury.
- By 2 weeks after SCI, 12% of patients have below-level neuropathic pain which is 'central'; by 6 months, 20% suffer central pain. However, the mean onset time is 1.8 ± 1.7 years (wide variation).
- The pathophysiology of central post-stroke pain (CPSP) involves a key role for lesions in diverse areas of the brain, including several different thalamic nuclei. One such lesion results in disinhibition of a nociceptive pathway that projects to the anterior cingulated cortex (limbic system) – this pathophysiology is associated with the burning quality of CPSP.
- The pathophysiology of SCI pain involves a 'spinal generator' and a 'supraspinal generator/amplifier'.
- Treatment of central pain is extremely challenging and requires a multimodal approach based on a biopsychosocial model. Differential diagnosis of pain type is crucial. New innovative physical/psychological treatments show promise of addressing maladaptive brain neuroplasticity changes.

- Pharmacotherapy is based on only a small number of controlled studies that demonstrate efficacy of amitriptyline for CPSP and pregabalin in both SCI and CPSP. Short-term efficacy has been reported for systemic (intravenous infusion) lidocaine (lignocaine), propofol and ketamine. However, there is no evidence of long-term efficacy.
- Dorsal root entry zone lesioning can provide long-term relief of central pain after brachial plexus avulsion.

Key references

Andersen G, Vestergaard K, Ingeman-Nielsen M, Jensen TS. Incidence of central post-stroke pain. *Pain* 1995;61:187–93.

Finnerup NB, Treatment of central pain. In: Castro-Lopec J, Rajas S, Schmelz M, eds. *Pain 2008. An Updated Review. Refresher Course Syllabus.* Seattle: IASP Press, 2008:319–26.

Gustin SM, Wrigley PJ, Gandevia SC et al. Movement imagery increases pain in people with neuropathic pain following complete thoracic spinal cord injury. *Pain* 2008;137:237–44.

Henry JL, Panju A, Yashpal K, eds. *Central Neuropathic Pain: Focus on Post-Stroke Pain.* Seattle: IASP Press, 2007.

Hocking G, Cousins MJ. Ketamine in chronic pain management: an evidence-based review. *Anesth Analg* 2003;97:1730–9.

Siddall PJ, Cousins MJ, Otte A et al. Pregabalin in central neuropathic pain associated with spinal cord injury: a placebo-controlled trial. *Neurology* 2006;67:1792–800.

Siddall PJ, McClelland JM, Rutkowski SB, Cousins MJ. A longitudinal study of the prevalence and characteristics of pain in the first 5 years following spinal cord injury. *Pain* 2003;103:249–57.

Siddall PJ, Molloy AR, Walker S et al. The efficacy of intrathecal morphine and clonidine in the treatment of pain after spinal cord injury. *Anesth Analg* 2000;91: 1493–8.

Siddall PJ, Yezierski RP, Loeser JD. Taxonomy and epidemiology of spinal cord injury pain. In: Yezierski RP, Burchiel K, eds. *Spinal Cord Injury Pain: Assessment, Mechanisms, Management. Progress in Pain Research and Management Vol 23.* Seattle: IASP Press, 2002:9–24.

Yezierski RP. Spinal cord injury: a model for the pathophysiology and mechanisms of central pain. In: Castro-Lopec J, Rajas S, Schmelz M, eds. *Pain 2008. An Updated Review. Refresher Course Syllabus.* Seattle: IASP Press, 2008:307–17.

Persistent postsurgical pain

It is now clear from numerous studies that persistent postsurgical pain (PPSP) is one of the major causes of persistent (chronic) pain. Limited data also indicate that a significant percentage of patients continue to have pain following trauma, particularly trauma to multiple body areas or traumatic amputation.

Pathophysiology

Although there is evidence that nerve damage plays a key role, there are other factors that probably determine which patients with nerve damage progress from acute to persistent pain as, in many operations (e.g. amputation), all patients have nerve damage but only a percentage (10–50%) progress to chronic pain (Table 7.1). The only reliable data currently available derive from postsurgery patients and thus this discussion will be limited to these patients. It is possible, but not studied, that similar factors may occur in post-trauma patients

TABLE 7.1

Estimated incidence of persistent postsurgical pain following selected procedures

Procedure	Incidence of PPSP (%)
Amputation	30–50
Thoracotomy	20–50
Mastectomy	10–30
Major joint replacement	12
Hysterectomy	5–32
Inguinal hernia repair	5–10
Cesarean section	5–10

PPSP, persistent postsurgical pain.

(many of whom also undergo surgery). A major review of this subject by Kehlet et al. was published in 2006.

The factors in Table 7.2 are associated with increased risk of PPSP, but no comprehensive study has been carried out to evaluate their relative importance. Although evidence of genetic factors is not

---

TABLE 7.2

Factors contributing to the development of persistent postsurgical pain

Pre-existing pain
- Central nervous system hyperexcitability
- Opioid tolerance

Physical nerve injury
- Location of surgical procedure (for example, chest wall)
- Surgical technique

Postoperative pain severity
- Inadequate analgesia techniques
- Extent of tissue injury
- Psychological factors (for example, depression)
- Sex
- Genetics including pharmacogenetics

Impaired nerve repair (or aggravated injury)
- Radiotherapy
- Chemotherapy

Other factors
- Genetic
- Psychological

From Macintyre P, Scott DA. Acute pain management and acute pain services. In: Cousins et al., 2009 (see Useful resources).

available for PPSP, Tegeder et al. (2006) have identified a genetic influence on the development of chronic pain following an acute episode of sciatica.

Prevention

Preoperative pain intensity has been correlated with postoperative pain intensity in a prospective study of 346 patients undergoing abdominal surgery. The intensity of postoperative pain has been linked to the prevalence of chronic pain. Thus, improved acute pain control pre- and postoperatively may help to prevent PPSP. There is also evidence that intra- and postoperative use of epidural neural blockade may be helpful. Surgical technique may play a role, as 'nerve preservation' techniques appear to lower incidence of PPSP – although no studies have prospectively addressed this area. The introduction of video-assisted thoracic surgery made no difference to the incidence of post-thoracotomy PPSP at 1 year after surgery. This serves to illustrate how difficult it is to avoid trauma to nerves at various surgical sites, and that factors other than nerve injury are involved in PPSP.

Treatment

In the early stages of PPSP surgeons tend to suspect a surgical complication of some sort (e.g. a wound hematoma, chronic infection, incomplete repair of an inguinal hernia). Initially, a reasonable attempt should be made to rule out such diagnoses. However, in the majority of cases no remediable surgical complication will be found. Recognition that the patient has chronic pain, and that the pathophysiology is in the central nervous system, not in the peripheral tissues, is now needed.

As the majority of PPSP is caused by nerve damage the treatment options are similar to those for other neuropathic pain syndromes. Pharmacotherapy alone will rarely be sufficient. A biopsychosocial assessment should be made and treatment plans should aim to rectify maladaptive changes in physical, psychological and environmental domains. For example, patients are rarely told that PPSP is a possible complication of surgery. Thus, patients often feel angry and let down and find it difficult to move on unless the anger is addressed with careful explanation and reassurance. Patients may have been stigmatized at work because of a perceived unnecessarily long recovery, requiring input to the workplace. In our experience patients with PPSP often have substantial contributions to their pain from psychosocial factors and this is borne out by several studies.

Pharmacotherapy relies on tricyclic antidepressants, anticonvulsants and sometimes membrane stabilizers. In severe cases a trial of subcutaneous peripheral nerve stimulation (PNS) may be necessary. PNS is emerging as a valuable option for postinguinal hernia repair PPSP. In a trial stimulation, electrodes are placed across the path of ilio-inguinal, iliohypogastric and genitofemoral nerves; if the trial stimulation is successful patients proceed at a later date to implantation of electrodes and pulse generator.

Postincisional pain

Postincisional syndrome is defined as pain at or close to the site of a surgical incision that persists beyond the usual healing period. As with other neuropathic pain syndromes, patients exhibit allodynia and sometimes also edema in the vicinity of the surgical wound.

Postamputation persistent pain

Postamputation persistent pain is a special case of PPSP because large nerves are deliberately cut in all patients. It is interesting, then, that only 30–50% develop PPSP, whereas 100% have nerve injury (see Table 7.1). This emphasizes the multifactorial basis of PPSP. A surprising omission in studies of amputation pain is information about how the nerves amputated are managed (i.e. clean cut or ligature tied). Use of a ligature tie in animal studies is known to generate neuropathic pain.

The clinical context of amputation may play a role. For example, when the amputation occurs because of a progressive disease, such as diabetes, disease-related preoperative nerve damage and pain are involved. Conversely, traumatic amputation or amputation to prevent spread of disease, such as in breast cancer, may not involve prior nerve damage or pain.

Pathophysiology. The neuromas that form at the end of cut nerves after amputation are hypersensitive and have abnormally dense

87

sodium (and other ion) channels that generate ectopic discharges. This abnormal activity initiates and maintains the central sensitization associated with nerve injury (see Chapter 1). There may also be a change in the distribution of sodium channel subtypes, with an upregulation of $Na_V1.8$. This opens up a possible new selective target, as $Na_V1.8$ occurs only on small primary afferent fibers. As with central pain, after amputation there is synaptic reorganization in the spinal cord, brainstem, thalamus and primary somatosensory cortex, which becomes newly responsive to neighboring body parts. These changes contribute to the persistent pain experienced after amputation.

Diagnosis. Phantom experiences, phantom pain and stump pain are different entities that share the same pathophysiological mechanisms. A phantom experience is a non-painful sensation; phantom pain is pain in an absent body part; and stump pain is local pain in the residual limb (i.e. at the amputation site). Up to 96% of amputees report phantom experiences, and 49% complain of stump pain. Depending on the tissue amputated, phantom pain may have an early prevalence in excess of 50%. Phantom pain affects not only limbs; phantom bladder, rectal, penile, breast and vaginal pain after surgery are all well described.

While phantom sensations may be described as tingling or itchy, phantom pain consists primarily of burning, cramping and shooting pains. Phantom sensations and phantom pain typically begin within days of the amputation, and tend to decrease in frequency and duration over time, though they persist for years in 40% of amputees. Sometimes phantom pain in the missing body part is similar to the pain present before the amputation.

Prevention. To date, attempts to prevent the development of phantom pain using peridural anesthesia or regional blocks have not proven successful. However, the randomized controlled trials (RCTs) that have evaluated these preventive regimens have not uniformly suppressed afferent input from the involved site. Therefore, the results of the studies should be interpreted as inconclusive rather than negative.

Key points – persistent postsurgical pain

- Persistent postsurgical pain (PPSP) is defined as pain at or close to the site of surgical incision that persists beyond the expected healing period.
- The incidence of PPSP varies from about 10% for very limited peripheral surgery, such as inguinal hernia repair or joint replacement, to 10–30% for mastectomy and up to 50% for thoracotomy and amputation.
- Nerve injury plays an important role in pathogenesis, but genetics, pre-existing pain and severity of postoperative pain are also risk factors, in addition to cancer treatment and possible psychosocial factors.
- Effective acute pain control may be preventive for PPSP – for example, intra- and postoperative use of epidural analgesia can prevent PPSP following some operations.
- Pharmacotherapy is based on results of studies of neuropathic drugs for treatment of pain due to other types of nerve injury. Tricyclic antidepressants and anticonvulsants are first-line drugs.
- Peripheral nerve stimulation is emerging as a possible option for severe PPSP.

Treatment

Ketamine, a non-competitive N-methyl D-aspartate (NMDA) receptor antagonist, has been used in humans to treat various neuropathic pain syndromes. Intravenous ketamine provides relief from phantom and stump pain, but one small crossover RCT indicated a high incidence of side effects.

Opioids. Small randomized studies have suggested that morphine decreases pain intensity, albeit during short-term observation periods.

Antidepressants and anticonvulsants. There is a scarcity of controlled trial results to guide clinicians in the treatment of phantom pain, and clinicians must rely on favorable results from clinical research in which these agents have been given to treat other neuropathic pain syndromes.

Mirror therapy, which is based on manipulating neuroplastic changes in the brain associated with phantom pain, has been reported to reduce phantom limb pain in clinical reports and in a small RCT in which it was significantly more effective ($p = 0.008$) for reducing pain than guided imagery and sham mirror therapy.

Neurostimulation of various types (low- and high-intensity transcutaneous electrical nerve stimulation [TENS], transcranial magnetic stimulation of the motor cortex, epidural cervical spinal cord simulation and epidural motor cortex stimulation) has been reported to be effective for phantom pain in case series, though carefully controlled trials have yet to be performed.

Key references

Aasvang EK, Brandsborg B, Christensen B et al. Neurophysiological characterization of postherniotomy pain. *Pain* 2008;137:173–81.

Aasvang E, Kehlet H. Chronic postoperative pain: the case of inguinal herniorrhaphy. *Br J Anaesth* 2005;95:69–76.

Brandsborg B, Nikolajsen L, Hansen CT et al. Risk factors for chronic pain after hysterectomy: a nationwide questionnaire and database study. *Anesthesiology* 2007;106:1003–12.

Brennan TJ, Kehlet H. Preventive analgesia to reduce wound hyperalgesia and persistent postsurgical pain: not an easy path. *Anesthesiology* 2005;103:681–3.

Bruce J, Drury N, Poobalan AS et al. The prevalence of chronic chest and leg pain following cardiac surgery: a historical cohort study. *Pain* 2003;104:265–73.

Chan BL, Witt R, Charrow AP et al. Mirror therapy for phantom limb pain. *N Engl J Med* 2007;357:2206–7.

Cruccu G, Aziz TZ, Garcia-Larrea L et al. EFNS guidelines on neurostimulation therapy for neuropathic pain. *Eur J Neurol* 2007;14:952–70.

Jung BF, Ahrendt GM, Oaklander AL, Dworkin RH. Neuropathic pain following breast cancer surgery: proposed classification and research update. *Pain* 2003;104:1–13.

Kehlet H. Chronic pain after groin hernia repair. *Br J Surg* 2008;95:135–6.

Kehlet H, Jensen TS, Woolf CJ. Persistent postsurgical pain: risk factors and prevention. *Lancet* 2006;367:1618–25.

Nikolajsen L, Brandsborg B, Lucht U et al. Chronic pain following total hip arthroplasty: a nationwide questionnaire study. *Acta Anaesthesiol Scand* 2006;50:495–500.

Nikolajsen L, Sorensen HC, Jensen TS, Kehlet H. Chronic pain following Caesarean section. *Acta Anaesthesiol Scand* 2004;48:111–6.

Tegeder I, Costigan M, Griffin RS et al. GTP cyclohydrolase and tetrahydrobiopterin regulate pain sensitivity and persistence. *Nat Med* 2006;12:1269–77.

Young Casey C, Greenberg MA, Nicassio PM et al. Transition from acute to chronic pain and disability: a model including cognitive, affective, and trauma factors. *Pain* 2008;134:69–79.

Pain in patients with cancer may present as various types of pain at different stages of the patient's journey with cancer. Thus, the pain may comprise acute, recurrent or chronic presentations due to the cancer and/or its treatment. Assessment of pain in patients with cancer should be the same as in other patients with pain (see Chapter 2), so that the widest possible range of treatments can be considered, with the aim of optimal treatment. Other additional symptoms such as fatigue, nausea and insomnia are common and also require treatment. Also, patients with cancer may have pre-existing chronic pain that continues, in addition to cancer pain (Table 8.1). Some patients with aggressive tumors may have escalating (or 'crescendo') pain requiring optimum pain management options, and the needs of cancer

TABLE 8.1

Types of pain in patients with cancer

- Patients with acute cancer-related pain
  - associated with the diagnosis of cancer
  - associated with cancer therapy (surgery, chemotherapy or radiation)
- Patients with chronic cancer-related pain
  - associated with cancer progression
  - associated with cancer therapy (surgery, chemotherapy or radiation)
- Patients with pre-existing chronic pain and cancer-related pain
- Patients with a history of drug addiction and cancer-related pain
  - actively involved in illicit drug use
  - in methadone maintenance programs
  - with a history of drug abuse
- Dying patients with cancer-related pain

'survivors' – who live for many years with chronic pain and who are increasing in numbers – also need to be addressed. Finally, patients with cancer require particular strategies during the end of life stage. The choice of treatment options is based on similar considerations to those for patients with chronic non-cancer pain.

Unfortunately, the prevalence of pain is high in cancer patients: 20–50% at time of diagnosis; 50% during treatment phase; 75–90% during the advanced cancer phase. At all of these stages still less than 50% of patients receive effective pain relief in studies in the USA, France and China – despite the fact that use of the *full range* of currently available options could provide relief for over 90% of patients. Sadly, this lamentable situation is no better for children, with a study in Australia in 2010 reporting that treatment was successful in only 47% of children. Many studies report that unrelieved cancer pain is associated with interference with several dimensions of quality of life of the patients and their carers. Prevalence and severity of pain may be lower in hematologic malignancies such as lymphomas and leukemias compared with solid tumors such as breast and prostate cancers, which commonly metastasize to bone. However, variability in presentation of pain and its treatment (see Tables 8.1 and 8.2) make it essential to carefully evaluate each patient regardless of the cancer type.

Pathophysiology

Acute pain occurs in cancer patients following surgery, radiotherapy or chemotherapy. After one or more of these treatments is finished, a percentage of patients progress to persistent pain (chronic pain). Risk factors in patients after cancer surgery are similar to those for any surgery (see Chapter 7, Table 7.2). The incidence of such pain is given in Table 7.1 (see page 84). It is likely that the risk of persistent pain is higher in patients who also receive radiotherapy and/or chemotherapy, in addition to surgery.

The large majority of episodes of acute cancer-related pain are due to tumor invasion of pain-sensitive structures, which causes pathophysiological processes of the 'injury response', including inflammation, edema, acidosis and necrosis. Specific pathophysiological mechanisms are shown in Table 8.2.

TABLE 8.2

Pain syndromes in patients with cancer: pain directly caused by cancer (primary or metastatic)

Mechanism	Characteristics of pain
Infiltration of bone by tumor ± fracture	Dull constant ache ± muscle spasm
Infiltration or compression of nerve tissue by tumor	Burning constant pain in area of sensory loss ± hyperalgesia ± paroxysmal pain
Obstruction of hollow viscus	Poorly localized dull deep sickening pain with superficial hyperalgesia over referred surface area
Occlusion of arteries and veins by tumor	Ischemic pain in skin or claudication (muscle) ± signs of ischemia or venous engorgement
Stretching of periosteum or fascia – in tissues with tight investment	Severe localized pain (periosteum) or typical visceral pain (e.g. ovary)
Inflammation, owing to necrosis and infection	Severe localized pain and signs of tumor infection (± superficial ulceration)
Soft tissue infiltration	Localized pain, foul-smelling if ulcerated
Raised intracranial pressure	Severe constant headache, confusion etc.
Spinal cord compression	Severe back pain – worse at night
	Subtle sensory changes initially, motor and sensory deficits eventually
	Urinary bladder control impaired

Many such pains improve with treatment of the cancer, but some will proceed to a chronic version of the acute presentation (Tables 8.2–8.5).

Chronic pain may be caused by the cancer, its treatment, conditions unrelated to the cancer (e.g. concurrent diseases) and/or factors in the psychosocial domains (see Tables 8.2–8.5). It is estimated that about

78% of pain is directly caused by the cancer, 19% by cancer treatment and 3% by concurrent diseases. However, many patients have multiple pain sites and pain types: for example, a high percentage (30–40%) have muscle pain in addition to cancer-related pain.

Diagnosing non-cancer pain is important as it emphasizes to patients the lack of a one-to-one relationship between the stage of cancer and the presence and severity of pain. However, Gonzales et al. (1991) found that, in 18% of patients presenting with pain as a problem, a thorough history and examination revealed new evidence of metastatic disease requiring anti-tumor treatment.

Metastatic spread of cancer to bone is the most common cause of cancer pain (Figure 8.1). Animal models using mice that had sarcoma cells implanted into the femur showed pain behavior related both to bone destruction and to the release of inflammatory mediators derived from the tumor (e.g. prostaglandins, cytokines, endothelins). Macrophages, which are often present in large numbers in some tumor

TABLE 8.3

Pain associated with cancer therapy

Mechanism	Examples
Following surgery	Acute postoperative pain
	Neuropathic pain due to nerve damage or amputation
Following radiotherapy	Acute nerve lesions
	Chronic radiation fibrosis causing nerve damage
	Myelopathy of spinal cord
	Peripheral nerve lesions
Following chemotherapy	Peripheral neuropathy in hands and feet
	Steroid-induced pseudo-rheumatism in multiple joints
	Aseptic necrosis due to steroids (in femoral or humoral head)
	Postherpetic neuralgia

TABLE 8.4

Pain from comorbid conditions

Mechanism	Common sites and pain characteristics
Neuropathy (e.g. diabetic)	Burning pain in hands, feet
Degenerative disk disease	Back pain ± radicular pain
Rheumatoid arthritis	Joint pain on movement
Diffuse osteoporosis	Back pain, limb pain
Posture abnormalities	Back pain, muscle spasm etc. with depression, after surgery etc.
Myofascial pain syndromes	Local muscle pain ± spasm
Headache	Tension type or migraine

masses, also produce mediators such as tumor necrosis factor and interleukins capable of activating nociceptors (see Chapter 1).

Yet chronic cancer pain is a nociceptive mosaic; pain may be due to tumor infiltration of nerves (neuropathic pain) or other tissues (somatic or visceral pain), or may be related to the treatment or procedure that the patient receives. Given the spectrum of potential pain sources and mechanisms, it is clear that several elements may be active in a single patient with cancer pain and that treatment should address all the pain mechanisms at play (Tables 8.2–8.5). Thus, regardless of the initial cause of pain, central sensitization can play a key role in cancer pain (see Chapter 1). Also neuroplastic changes may occur in the brain (see Chapter 1).

As with all chronic pain, psychosocial factors are of profound importance in patients with cancer pain (Table 8.5). Saunders' concept of 'total pain' encompasses all of the factors that may affect the pain experienced by patients with cancer, including physical, psychological, social and spiritual elements.

TABLE 8.5

Psychological comorbidities augmenting pain

Psychological factor	Possible causes
Anxiety	Sleeplessness
	Fear of death; loss of dignity (loss of self-control)
	Fear of surgical mutilation; uncontrollable pain
	Fear of the future; loss of social position and work
	Confused understanding of disease owing to poor communication
	Family and financial problems
Depression	Sleeplessness
	Loss of physical abilities
	Sense of helplessness
	Disfigurement
	Loss of valued social position, financial problems
Anger	Frustration with therapeutic failures
	Resentment of sickness
	Irritability caused by pain and general discomfort

A vicious circle usually develops:

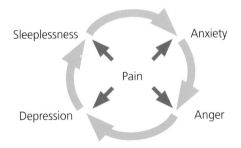

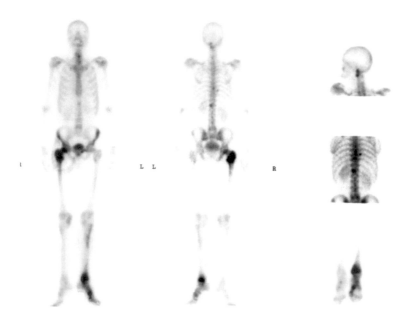

Figure 8.1 Bone scintigraphy of a 54-year-old man with prostate cancer and bone metastases. The scans show increased uptake at the sites of metastases in the cervical and lumbar spine, femur, tibia and metatarsal bone.

Assessment

The same principles of pain assessment as described in Chapter 2 apply to patients with cancer pain. However, in this scenario, it is crucial to establish whether the pain is related to the cancer itself, the associated treatments or other conditions (see Tables 8.2–8.5). Thus, patients should be asked about the onset of pain – whether it was present before the cancer or associated with the initiation of treatments such as surgery, chemotherapy or radiotherapy – and whether it has progressed. An oncological history must be added to the general medical component of the patient's history. The findings of a new physical examination may suggest a relapse or the interim development of new metastases that would warrant further investigation, so CT scans, MRI and other investigations are more readily ordered in cancer patients.

Efforts should be made to identify the specific underlying pain syndrome, as the different types may respond differently to various analgesic therapies (Tables 8.1–8.5). In addition, open discussions with patients and their families about concerns and misconceptions surrounding the use of opioids should take place early on, as opioids are the treatment of choice for moderate to severe cancer pain.

Treatment

A comprehensive assessment (see Chapter 2) is essential in identifying the basis of the pain in individual cancer patients (Tables 8.2–8.5). The key to effective treatment of cancer pain lies in choosing from one or more options that are now available, rather than relying only on one option such as pharmacological management. This is particularly important for 'cancer survivors' with chronic pain. Many of the preceding chapters describe pain conditions and treatments that are applicable to cancer patients with chronic pain, with treatments in the areas of: pharmacology, physical therapy, psychological strategies, interventional treatments and other options.

Pharmacological management

Opioids are the foundation for management of cancer pain of moderate or severe intensity, especially opioids that are full agonists at the morphine receptor (e.g. morphine, oxycodone, hydromorphone). Partial agonist opioids (e.g. buprenorphine) exhibit a ceiling effect for analgesia as dose increases, although this analgesic ceiling is rarely reached at the usual clinical doses. Full opioid agonists do not show this ceiling effect.

Agonist–antagonist opioids also activate the κ-opioid receptor while simultaneously blocking the μ-opioid receptor, thereby risking precipitation of an opioid abstinence syndrome in patients already on a regimen of a full opioid agonist such as morphine. Therefore, only full opioid agonists at the morphine receptor should normally be used for cancer pain. The partial agonist buprenorphine, available as a skin patch, has emerged as an option for mild-to-moderate pain. Unlike agonist–antagonists it does not precipitate opioid abstinence syndrome, rather producing additive analgesic effects when used together with full opioid agonists.

Meperidine should be avoided in patients with cancer pain. Prolonged administration of this agent leads to accumulation of normeperidine, a toxic metabolite of meperidine with an approximate 20-hour half-life, which causes dysphoria and seizures.

Mechanism of action. Opioids hyperpolarize nociceptive cell membranes, shorten the duration of their action potentials and inhibit the release of excitatory mediators. All of these actions decrease nociceptive transmission and produce analgesia.

Effect size. Study results have shown that 1 of every 3 individuals taking morphine obtains substantial pain relief.

Adverse effects. Drowsiness, nausea, vomiting, urinary retention and pruritus are frequent side effects of opioids: 1 of every 3 previously opioid-naive individuals develops at least one of these side effects. The risk of respiratory depression when the opioid dose is carefully titrated to decrease cancer pain is less than 1% in the opioid-naive patient, although it is higher in older individuals. The risk of respiratory depression and all other opioid adverse effects – apart from constipation – decreases with chronic opioid administration. Constipation is almost universal during chronic opioid administration, so when chronic opioid therapy is started, a prophylactic 'bowel regimen' should also be initiated, comprising a stool softener and a stimulant cathartic. In some countries oxycodone and the opioid receptor antagonist naloxone are combined in an oral slow-release long-acting preparation. The naloxone has a local action on opioid receptors in the gut, thus preventing or ameliorating constipation. On the first pass through the liver most of the naloxone is metabolized.

Route of administration. Oral administration is the route of choice for chronic analgesia because of its convenience, safety, rapid onset and low cost. A systematic review of the literature has shown that the route of administration does not affect the degree of analgesia. Furthermore, controlled-release preparations are not superior to immediate-release forms in terms of pain relief or side effects, but are advantageous in terms of duration of analgesia – particularly at night.

Tolerance. Commonly, the pain-relieving effect of opioids is assumed to decline with repeated administration – that is, tolerance develops, as has been demonstrated in intact laboratory animals. Yet clinical experience indicates that tolerance to opioid analgesia is rarely the sole reason for dose escalation. The need for high doses of opioid from the start of therapy suggests an opioid-resistant pain mechanism (e.g. neuropathic pain). When abrupt dose escalation is needed, a physical reason is usually apparent (i.e. metastasis). In fact, in animal models of chronic inflammation, opioid analgesia does not decrease to any great extent during chronic exposure. Therefore, there are valid concerns about decisions to withhold opioids or to restrict necessary dose increases. Recent studies of the role of microglia (see Chapter 1, Figure 1.8) indicate that glial cell activation plays a role in development of opioid tolerance – as well as increasing pain via central sensitization. Thus, the use of glial-blocking drugs may play a future role in ameliorating opioid tolerance.

Opioid rotation. When the dose escalates to a level associated with unsatisfactory side effects and no physical reason is apparent, opioids should be 'rotated' – that is, the dose should be tapered and the opioid discontinued while another one is started. Cross-tolerance is only partial, and rotation enables clearance of metabolites such as morphine-3-glucuronide, a morphine metabolite. If uncleared, these metabolites could antagonize opioid analgesia.

Risk of addiction. Addiction is defined as the compulsive use of a substance that results in physical, psychological and social harm to the user and continued use of the substance despite such harm. The risk of addiction in patients receiving opioids for the first time for medical purposes, such as the treatment of cancer pain, is very low (see also Chapter 2).

Addiction is distinct from physical dependence, although the terms are sometimes inaccurately used interchangeably. Physical dependence is a biological phenomenon defined as the development of an abstinence syndrome following abrupt discontinuation of therapy or administration of an antagonist. Physical dependence may occur during chronic administration of many classes of drugs, including opioids, benzodiazepines, barbiturates, alcohol, β-blockers and the

α_2-agonist clonidine. Physical dependence is of little clinical importance as long as abrupt discontinuation of therapy is avoided. However, patients with addiction problems do develop cancer pain and require special management.

Breakthrough pain describes a typically brief episode of pain above a baseline pain intensity that is controlled by a long-acting or by-the-clock opioid. Treatment of breakthrough pain requires the use of rescue medication that offers a rapid onset of action and short duration. This allows patients to obtain prompt relief while avoiding lingering opioid effects once the pain intensity has returned to baseline. Short-acting oral opioids are used for this purpose. More rapid onset of analgesia can be obtained with oral transmucosal fentanyl (fentanyl lozenges), transbuccal fentanyl tablets or transnasal ketamine. Controlled trials have demonstrated the efficacy of these new options.

Non-steroidal anti-inflammatory drugs

Mechanism of action. Non-steroidal anti-inflammatory drugs (NSAIDs) decrease inflammation by inhibiting the synthesis of peripheral prostaglandins. NSAIDs also have central analgesic properties that are distinguishable from their peripheral anti-inflammatory effects. They inhibit prostaglandin synthesis in the spinal cord, modulate N-methyl D-aspartate receptor activity, activate descending inhibitory pain projections and hyperpolarize cell membranes. All of these actions decrease nociceptive transmission and produce analgesia. Apart from their effects on prostaglandins, NSAIDs also affect other processes such as nuclear transcription factors and ion (K^+) channel function.

Ceiling and dose-sparing effects. NSAIDs exhibit a ceiling effect for analgesia, and therefore should not be administered above the recommended dose range. At higher doses, there is no incremental analgesic benefit and the risk of side effects increases dramatically.

Consensus, reached after an advisory panel was convened to address the issue of cyclooxygenase-2 (COX-2) safety on the cardiac and cerebrovascular side effects of selective inhibitors of COX-2, has prompted withdrawal of rofecoxib and valdecoxib. Celecoxib remains on the market. Although this agent has been associated with an increased risk of cardiovascular events in a long-term placebo-controlled trial, chronic use of traditional NSAIDs, with the exception of ASA (aspirin), has also been associated with an increased risk of serious cardiovascular events. Patients in need of analgesics for chronic pain should therefore be informed of the risks, and the lowest effective doses should be prescribed for the shortest appropriate duration.

NSAIDs have an opioid-sparing effect, which can be harnessed for the relief of pain of moderate or severe intensity by starting the NSAID before, or at the same time as, an opioid. Clinical consensus is that the combination of an NSAID and an opioid augments pain relief by producing greater analgesia than that achieved with either drug individually. However, the results of meta-analyses question whether this benefit has been demonstrated in clinical trials.

Effect size. Meta-analyses of randomized controlled trials (RCTs) have shown that NSAIDs are effective for the treatment of cancer pain of mild intensity that does not originate from nerve damage. Trial findings have shown that 1 of every 3 individuals using ibuprofen and 1 of every 5 individuals using paracetamol (acetaminophen) obtain substantial pain relief.

Adverse effects. NSAID use is associated with risks of serious gastrointestinal bleeding, impaired renal function, exacerbation of hypertension or worsening of heart failure, and bleeding due to inhibition of platelet aggregation. Older patients have a particularly increased risk of serious gastrointestinal adverse effects after taking NSAIDs. Trials have shown that 1 of every 111 older patients receiving NSAIDs has serious gastrointestinal bleeding that would not have occurred otherwise.

Drugs used for treatment of neuropathic cancer pain. See pages 62–5 and 68–9 for discussion of anticonvulsants, antidepressants, corticosteroids, capsaicin, opioids and lidocaine (lignocaine) patches. Important 'third-line' treatments in cancer pain include low-dose ketamine infusion (150–500 µg/kg/hour) and/or lidocaine infusion (1–1.5 mg/kg/hour), either of which can be given intravenously or subcutaneously.

Bisphosphonates are analogs of pyrophosphates and are powerful inhibitors of bone resorption. Bisphosphonates are useful for the relief of pain due to bone metastases. A systematic review of the literature of RCTs, however, has shown that their effectiveness is only moderate at best, their analgesic effect is not immediate and their use is associated with frequent side effects. Therefore, they should not be considered as first-line therapy. At 4 weeks, 1 of every 11 individuals given bisphosphonates obtains substantial pain relief and 1 of every 16 patients discontinues the therapy because of side effects.

Non-pharmacological treatment

External radiotherapy employs ionizing radiation to destroy cancer cells. A systematic review of RCTs found that radiation is efficacious to treat pain from bone metastasis. The trial data indicate that 1 of every 4 individuals treated with external radiotherapy experiences 50% pain relief within 1 month.

Radiation therapy produces pain relief by inducing apoptotic death, not only of tumor cells, thereby reducing pressure in the bone marrow, but also of highly radiosensitive inflammatory cells. The multifraction regimen is the most widely used (i.e. 30 Gy delivered in ten treatment fractions over 2 weeks). However, no particular fractionation schedule has been found to be superior.

Radionuclide therapy is the systemic use of radioisotopes; it is a form of internal radiotherapy. Radioisotopes produce pain relief with a similar degree, onset and duration as radiotherapy. However, thrombocytopenia and neutropenia are common toxic effects of radioisotopes.

A systematic review of RCTs has found that a combination of strontium radioisotopes and radiotherapy produces better quality of life scores than radiotherapy alone.

Education, self-help, cognitive behavioral therapy and other options. Cancer patients benefit from the same range of treatment options that are used for chronic non-cancer pain. Treatments found to be effective include:

- patient education about pain and pain management, which improve pain, pain knowledge and attitudes, use of pain medication and interference by pain in activities of daily living
- self-help programs, which are supported by evidence in patients with chronic non-cancer pain
- cognitive behavioral therapy programs, which are successfully used in non-cancer pain and appear to be helpful in cancer patients
- hypnosis and relaxation strategies
- music therapy (beneficial in some patients).

Invasive procedures

Invasive options broadly consist of neurolytic (e.g. neurolytic celiac plexus block), neurodestructive (e.g. radiofrequency lesioning or neurosurgical anterolateral spinothalamic cordotomy) or neuromodulatory (e.g. intrathecal or epidural drug administration or spinal cord and peripheral nerve neurostimulation) procedures.

Neurolytic celiac plexus block. Visceral pain from upper abdominal viscera is initiated by noxious stimuli, for example due to cancer of the pancreas, transmitted via visceral nociceptive afferents which traverse the largest of the sympathetic plexuses (the celiac plexus) and thence reach the splanchnic nerves, dorsal root ganglia and spinal cord. Neurolytic block can be carried out at the level of the celiac plexus or splanchnic nerves. Both techniques have similar efficacy with 70–94% of patients receiving immediate good relief, which lasts until death in 75% of patients. However, the safety of the procedure relies on thorough knowledge of the anatomy, technique and potential complications (including paraplegia). The procedure is routinely carried out under guidance of fluoroscopy or CT scan.

An advantage of the splanchnic nerve approach is the much smaller volume required, thus permitting the use of 10% phenol mixed with contrast medium in a volume of 2–3 mL on each side – compared with up to 10–25 mL of absolute alcohol on each side for celiac plexus block. This aspect of the two procedures favors splanchnic block as hypotension is less likely (avoidance of lumbar sympathetic block) and paraplegia risk is reduced (smaller volume for spread onto spinal nerve roots and spinal cord). However, splanchnic block requires placement of the needles one spinal segment higher than for celiac block – thus increasing the risk of pneumothorax. Burton et al. have published a detailed evaluation of risks and benefits.

Other neurolytic procedures such as intrathecal alcohol or phenol are now rarely used because of the greater flexibility and lower risk of side effects of intraspinal drug administration.

Neurodestructive neurosurgical procedures are now much less frequently used for pain directly related to cancer, because of the availability of intraspinal drug administration (ISDA). However, it is rare for ISDA to completely relieve cancer pain, whereas anterolateral spinothalamic cordotomy can produce such a result lasting up to a year or more. For example, cordotomy can be an important option for patients with intrapelvic cancer involving soft tissues and the lumbosacral plexus, as such patients have severe refractory pain and often have a long life expectancy. However, after variable periods of time pain may develop on the opposite side of the body (mirror image pain), due to an alternative ipsilateral spinothalamic tract. This procedure requires considerable skill and experience and few centers currently have this expertise.

Radiofrequency lesioning. Cancer patients frequently have co-morbidities such as back pain due to degenerative spinal disease. Such problems may be amenable to radiofrequency lesioning.

Intraspinal drug administration has emerged as the most frequently used invasive procedure for cancer pain that is unresponsive to multimodal systemic pharmacological treatment and other non-invasive treatments. The efficacy of ISDA has been confirmed in a randomized clinical trial. Many drugs other than opioids are now used for ISDA in an approach termed 'spinal analgesic chemotherapy' (see Carr and Cousins 2009) to respond to various types, locations and severity of cancer pain. The most frequently used ISDA system is a percutaneous intrathecal catheter; however, epidural systems can be useful if local anesthesia is to be used for pain that is well localized (e.g. for mesothelioma-related chest wall pain). Fully implanted programmable pumps can be used for patients with a longer-term prognosis.

Neurostimulation techniques are invaluable for treatment of neuropathic pain such as post-mastectomy neuralgia, intractable migraine and other conditions.

Key points – cancer pain

- Cancer pain is a nociceptive mosaic in which pain may arise from inflammation, tumor infiltration of nerves (neuropathic pain) or other tissues (visceral or somatic pain), treatment, diagnostic and therapeutic procedures, and from other psychological and environmental factors.
- Non-steroidal anti-inflammatory drugs exhibit a ceiling effect for analgesia and should not be administered above the recommended dose.
- Opioids are the foundation for management of cancer pain of moderate to severe intensity.
- Oral administration is the route of choice for chronic analgesia unless it is ineffective or contraindicated, or the patient prefers another route.
- Treatment of breakthrough pain requires the use of rescue medication with a rapid onset and short duration of action.
- Meperidine and mixed agonist–antagonist opioids should be avoided in patients with cancer pain.
- Radiotherapy is effective for pain from bone metastases.
- Neurolytic celiac plexus block decreases pain intensity in patients with inoperable pancreatic cancer.
- Spinal opioid and non-opioid drug administration is an effective flexible method for patients for whom systemic drug administration has failed or who suffer intolerable side effects with such treatment.

Key references

American Pain Society. *Guideline for the Management of Cancer Pain in Adults and Children.* Illinois: American Pain Society, 2006. www.ampainsoc.org/pub/cancer.htm, last accessed 4 Nov 2010.

American Pain Society. *Principles of Analgesic Use in the Treatment of Acute Pain and Cancer Pain.* 5th edn. Illinois: American Pain Society, 2006. www.ampainsoc.org/pub/principles. htm, last accessed 4 Nov 2010.

Bennett MI, Bagnall AM, Jose Closs S. How effective are patient-based educational interventions in the management of cancer pain? Systematic review and meta-analysis. *Pain* 2009;143:192–9.

Burton AW, Phan PC, Cousins MJ. In: Cousins et al., 2009 (see Useful resources).

Carr DB, Cousins MJ. In: Cousins et al., 2009 (see Useful resources).

Carr DB, Goudas LC, Balk EM et al. Evidence report on the treatment of pain in cancer patients. *J Natl Cancer Inst Monogr* 2004:23–31.

Gonzales GR, Elliott KJ, Portenoy RK, Foley KM. The impact of a comprehensive evaluation in the management of cancer pain. *Pain* 1991;47:141–4.

Jacox AK, Carr DB, Payne R et al. *Management of Cancer Pain. Clinical Practice Guidelines.* AHCPR Publication No 94-0595. Maryland: Agency for Health Care Policy and Research, 1994.

McNicol E, Strassels SA, Goudas L et al. NSAIDS or paracetamol, alone or combined with opioids, for cancer pain. *Cochrane Database Syst Rev* 2005, issue 2. CD005180. www.thecochranelibrary.com.

McQuay HJ, Carroll D, Moore RA. Radiotherapy for painful bone metastases: a systematic review. *Clin Oncol (R Coll Radiol)* 1997;9:150–4.

Niv D, Gofeld M. In: Cousins et al., 2009 (see Useful resources).

Prager JP, Stanton-Hicks M. In: Cousins et al., 2009 (see Useful resources).

Smith TJ, Coyne PJ, Staats PS et al. An implantable drug delivery system (IDDS) for refractory cancer pain provides sustained pain control, less drug-related toxicity, and possibly better survival compared with comprehensive medical management (CMM). *Ann Oncol* 2005;16:825–33.

Wolfe J, Grier HE, Klar N et al. Symptoms and suffering at the end of life in children with cancer. *N Engl J Med* 2000;342:326–33.

Wong R, Wiffen PJ. Bisphosphonates for the relief of pain secondary to bone metastases. *Cochrane Database Syst Rev* 2002, issue 2. CD002068. www.thecochranelibrary.com.

Yates P, Edwards H, Nash R et al. A randomized controlled trial of a nurse-administered educational intervention for improving cancer pain management in ambulatory settings. *Patient Educ Couns* 2004;53:227–37.

Chronic low back pain

Chronic back pain is defined by orthopedic surgeons as back pain that lasts longer than 7–12 weeks. Frequent recurring back pain is also classified as chronic pain, as it intermittently affects an individual over a long period. Chronic back pain has also been defined as pain that lasts beyond the expected period of healing. Furthermore, insurance and industrial sources consider individuals to have chronic back pain if their symptoms result in loss of work or disability.

Given this variety of definitions, estimates of prevalence vary (Table 9.1). In contrast to the prevalence of osteoarthritis (see pages 125–6), that of back pain decreases with age (Table 9.1). One epidemiological study in the Netherlands found that as many as 25% of individuals with new-onset low back pain were symptomatic at 12 months, though in most cases pain resolved within 2 months. Symptoms of pain in the lower back are more prevalent than those in the mid or upper back.

Pathophysiology. Chronic low back pain is a complex biopsychosocial process that cannot be explained on purely anatomic, biomechanical, neurophysiological, immunologic, inflammatory or neurochemical

TABLE 9.1

Estimates of prevalence for chronic low back pain

Prevalence	Range (%)
Point	12–33
1 year	22–65
Lifetime	11–84
In people aged < 80 years	14–51
In people aged ≥ 80 years	7–22

grounds. For example, job dissatisfaction and fear of re-injury are strong risk factors for the development of chronic pain in individuals with acute back pain. Low income and poor education are also risk factors for chronic back pain and disability. For these reasons some researchers argue that chronic disability from back pain is primarily related to a psychosocial dysfunction, but the validity and reliability of this statement is uncertain.

Models of low back pain indicate that mechanical and neurochemical factors interact closely. Mechanical trauma could lead to the production of metalloproteinases and cytokines; the actions of these substances on the extracellular matrix of the intervertebral disk produce disk degeneration and pain.

When the etiology of low back pain is apparent, there is most often a musculoskeletal abnormality of the lumbar spine, such as muscle strain, arthritis or disk degeneration or facet joint arthropathy. Back pain may also be accompanied by radiating pain in a radicular pattern into the lower limb due to nerve root irritation or compression (often called 'sciatica'). Low back pain may also be referred from visceral pathology, including vascular problems such as abdominal aortic aneurysm.

Like other chronic pain syndromes, chronic back pain may also involve central neuroplastic changes such as neuronal hyperactivity, changes in membrane excitability and expression of new genes that perpetuate pain even in the absence of new tissue injury.

Diagnosis. The diagnosis of chronic back pain is a clinical one. Although anatomic abnormalities can be readily identified by imaging studies, there is no causal relationship between radiographic findings and non-specific low back pain, because most radiological abnormalities are common in asymptomatic people. Reaching a specific diagnosis is often impossible.

The diagnostic strategy recommended by the US Agency for Healthcare Policy and Research in 1994 (now the Agency for Healthcare Research and Quality) remains valid today. It is appropriate to start symptomatic therapy without imaging in adults under 50 years of age who lack so-called 'red flags' – signs or symptoms of systemic disease or progressive neurological dysfunction indicating tumor, abscess, fracture or cauda equina syndrome.

For patients over 50 years of age, or for those whose history or physical findings raise the possibility of 'red flags', plain radiography and simple laboratory tests can almost completely rule out any serious underlying conditions such as fracture, cancer or abscess.

Indications for MRI or CT are shown in Table 9.2. Although physicians and patients prefer MRI to radiographic evaluations, MRI offers little additional benefit to patients. In fact, the use of MRI may elevate the costs of care because of the increased number of unnecessary spine operations.

If pain is not substantially improved within 6 weeks, further diagnostic evaluation is appropriate; the choice of imaging study depends on the clinical syndrome. Although MRI is a logical next step, CT scanning is less expensive and almost as accurate in identifying most underlying conditions, making it a reasonable alternative.

Preventive treatment

Exercise. A systematic review of randomized controlled trials (RCTs) has found that exercise and physical activity are of moderate utility for the prevention of chronic back pain.

Lumbar supports and back schools. There is strong evidence from RCTs that lumbar supports and back schools are not effective pre-emptive interventions. A back school is a structured educational

TABLE 9.2

Indications for MRI or CT in patients with back pain

• Major trauma	• Immunosuppression
• Age > 50 years	• Saddle anesthesia*
• History of cancer	• Bowel or bladder incontinence
• Unexplained weight loss	• Severe or progressive neurological deficit
• Fever	

*A physical symptom of numbness in the area of the buttocks and upper inner thighs, consistent with the portion of the body that would come into contact with a saddle.

program, usually in a group setting, designed to inform patients about low back problems.

Smoking and weight reduction. Smoking and excess weight are predictors of back pain. Although there is no persuasive evidence that modifying these risk factors relieves pain, most experts who take a comprehensive disease management and rehabilitation approach to back pain advise and prescribe weight reduction to reduce mechanical load on the spine combined with exercise and cognitive behavioral therapy (CBT).

Non-pharmacological treatment

Exercise. As with the findings for acute back pain, in which a return to usual activity is the most effective therapy, meta-analyses of RCTs have shown that exercise programs reduce pain and improve function in patients with subacute, chronic or persistent postsurgical low back pain. Supervised stretching and strengthening fitness programs achieve the largest improvement compared with unsupervised exercise. One RCT has found that lumbar flexion in the early morning (i.e. a form of self-care) reduces pain intensity and costs associated with chronic non-specific low back pain.

Massage and spinal manipulation. A meta-analysis of trials that evaluated massage has concluded that the technique is beneficial for subacute and chronic back pain. Methodological flaws in the analysed trials (lack of randomization or blinding) weaken the findings. Systematic reviews and a large RCT of 1334 participants have concluded that spinal manipulation produces a small-to-moderate benefit at 3 months; however, its effectiveness decreases over time and at 12 months the benefit is only small.

A separate meta-analysis concluded that spinal manipulation does not reduce neck pain; moreover, case reports have documented rare but serious cerebrovascular events due to arterial damage induced by cervical manipulation.

Acupuncture. A recent meta-analysis has indicated that acupuncture produces both short-term (6 weeks) and long-term (6 months) relief of chronic back pain even when sham acupuncture is used as a comparator. However, the available data are insufficient to compare the effectiveness of acupuncture with pharmacotherapy or non-drug therapies. Acupuncture is generally safe when compared with pharmacotherapy and other procedures.

CBT. A meta-analysis of RCTs has indicated that cognitive therapy reduces both pain intensity and behavioral expression of pain in patients with chronic pain (including those with back pain).

Other treatments. According to systematic reviews of the literature, transcutaneous electrical nerve stimulation (TENS) and the use of special corsets lack effectiveness for chronic back pain. However, they are often used as part of a comprehensive multimodal approach despite the lack of evidence to support such practice.

Pharmacological management

Non-steroidal anti-inflammatory drugs. Although non-steroidal anti-inflammatory drugs (NSAIDs) are effective for short-term symptomatic relief of acute low back pain, a systematic review found insufficient evidence to support their use for chronic low back pain.

RCTs that evaluate the combination of paracetamol (acetaminophen) plus weak opioids such as codeine or tramadol have found that these combinations reduce pain intensity. However, long-term effectiveness is unknown because of the short duration of the studies and the likelihood that tolerance would diminish the apparent analgesic benefit of such combinations during long-term clinical use.

Antidepressants. A systematic review of RCTs suggests that while antidepressants reduce the severity of chronic back pain, they do not improve functional status. As the comorbidity of depression may be quite high (15–80%) in those with chronic low back pain, particularly those treated at referral centers such as pain clinics, diagnosing depression and treating it appropriately is key to the successful treatment of back pain itself. Untreated depression reduces the positive impact of all back pain treatments.

Invasive treatment

Epidural steroid injections should not be used for non-specific low back pain; rather, their role is in treatment of back pain accompanied by radicular pain. Injections can be made either translaminar via a

113

posterior approach via the ligamentum flavum, or transforaminal via an oblique approach. Both techniques are best carried out with an image intensifier or CT control. In the acute phase of spinal nerve root irritation, early evidence points to the potential of transforaminal injection to prevent progression to chronic sciatica. However, rigorous controlled studies are not available. Of 8 patients who receive epidural steroid injections, 1 will experience at least 75% pain relief in the short term, but this benefit fades over time as only 1 out of 13 patients has 50% pain relief in the long term (12 weeks to 1 year).

Lumbar facet joint injections, medial branch blocks and radiofrequency lesioning. About 10–15% of patients with low back pain have at least part of their pain arising from the facet joints. Such patients may gain temporary relief from injection of local anesthesia and cortisone directly into the facet joint. Alternatively, the medial branch of the dorsal ramus of the appropriate spinal nerves can be blocked to provide potential temporary pain relief. This may be followed by radiofrequency lesioning to provide relief for about 6–12 months.

Such procedures do not cure back pain but may allow patients to move on to 'stretch and strengthen' programs, CBT and other options (see above).

Spinal cord stimulation is increasingly used for the treatment of chronic back pain, particularly in patients with failed spinal surgery syndrome (persistent pain and functional limitation after spinal surgery). A small RCT reported that patients with spinal cord stimulation were less likely to undergo reoperation. However, the value of this outcome is difficult to interpret as function and employment status were similar in both randomized groups after treatment.

Surgical treatment. Prospective cohort studies and RCTs have shown that, for patients with moderate to severe sciatica, surgical treatment yields greater short-term improvement than non-surgical treatment. On the other hand, conservative therapies should be considered the first line of treatment, as selecting a conservative treatment does not run the risk of surgical complications and the relative short-term benefit of surgery decreases over time.

There is no evidence that spinal fusion, one of the most common operations for low back problems, is superior to other surgical procedures such as laminectomy for common degenerative conditions of the spine. Interestingly, the outcome of spinal stenosis surgery does not seem to correlate with the degree of postsurgical spinal canal narrowing.

Interdisciplinary rehabilitation. Treatment designed to integrate several modalities that address the biopsychosocial factors perpetuating functional loss in chronic back pain, rather than attempting to find and treat a single cause (i.e. the 'pain generator'), is more effective for enabling patients disabled by low back pain to return to work and stay at work than are conventional or surgical treatments. Selectively combining treatments that, based on a biopsychosocial formulation, specifically address the perpetuating factor influencing recovery, appears to have the best chance of returning disabled patients to a functional quality of life.

Future treatment. Recently an 'artificial disk' has been approved for marketing, with the goal of preserving relatively normal spine architecture and mechanics after operations involving shrunken or extruded disks. Use of gene therapy such as adenovirus-mediated gene transfer to nucleus pulposus cells to halt or slow disk degeneration is also an attractive prospect.

Spinal stenosis

Spinal stenosis refers to congenital (rare) or acquired (common with advanced age) narrowing of the spinal canal or the foramina through which the nerve roots exit (Figure 9.1). Five in every 1000 people over 50 are estimated to have symptoms of spinal stenosis.

Pathophysiology. Typically, the condition occurs in the cervical or lumbar spine as a result of invasion of the spinal canal by osteophytes, tissue from hypertrophied facets, bulging disks and/or hypertrophy of the ligamentum flavum, the ligament that connects the laminae of the vertebrae and prevents excessive motion between the vertebral bodies.

(a)   (b)

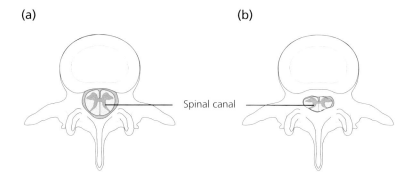

Figure 9.1 Cross-section of a vertebra with (a) a normal spinal canal and (b) stenosis of the canal and associated nerve compression.

Compression of the medullary and lumbar cord or nerve roots produces symptoms of chronic neck or back pain along with cervical or lumbar radiculopathy, respectively.

Diagnosis. Patients with spinal stenosis experience numbness, weakness of the extremities and (for lumbar stenosis) leg pain upon walking. The last symptom, termed 'neurogenic' claudication, occurs because, when the patient walks erect, increased epidural, intrathecal and foraminal pressures compromise microcirculation to the spinal cord and nerve roots. Patients with leg pain upon walking as a result of inadequate blood flow to one or both legs are said to have 'vascular' claudication.

Symptoms of lumbar stenosis typically occur on standing or walking down stairs, and improve when the patient leans forward (e.g. on a shopping cart in a supermarket). Leaning forward (or simply sitting down) tends to create more space in the spinal canal and foramina, thereby decreasing compression of neural tissue and the local blood supply that feeds it.

Treatment of spinal stenosis follows the same principles as described above for back pain, with the exception of one type of spinal stenosis termed 'cauda equina syndrome', which requires immediate surgical decompression. The cauda equina is so named because of the resemblance of the nerve roots at the caudal end of the spinal cord, which float freely within spinal fluid, to the tail of a horse.

Cauda equina syndrome is seen when severe pressure on the nerve fibers at the base of the spinal column results in loss of control of the bowel or bladder, pain, severe weakness, or loss of feeling in one or both legs. Immediate surgical decompression is indicated to relieve the pressure and prevent irreversible loss of spinal cord function. Additionally, high-dose glucocorticoids are indicated when the cause is inoperable cancer.

Key points – chronic low back pain and spinal stenosis

- When the etiology of low back pain is apparent, it is most often a musculoskeletal abnormality of the lumbar spine; however, low back pain may also be referred from visceral pathology.
- Chronic low back pain is a complex biopsychosocial process that cannot be explained on purely anatomic, biomechanical, neurophysiological, immunologic, inflammatory or neurochemical grounds.
- Symptomatic therapy can be initiated without imaging tests in adults under 50 who lack 'red flags' – history of major trauma, cancer, or signs or symptoms of systemic disease, tumor, immunocompromise, fracture, abscess, progressive and severe neurological loss, or cauda equina syndrome.
- For patients over 50 and those whose findings suggest systemic disease, plain radiography and simple laboratory tests can almost completely rule out underlying systemic disease.
- CT or MRI should be reserved for patients over 50 and those with 'red flags' (see above).
- Exercise has moderate utility in the prevention or treatment of chronic back pain.
- Pregabalin has small to modest analgesic efficacy
- Massage, spinal manipulation and acupuncture provide small-to-moderate short-term benefits.

- There is insufficient evidence to support the long-term use of non-steroidal anti-inflammatory drugs for the treatment of chronic low back pain, particularly in light of the increased risks for gastrointestinal bleeding and cardiovascular events.
- Epidural steroid injections produce small-to-moderate short-term pain relief.
- Antidepressants reduce pain severity but do not improve function.
- Integrated treatments that address the salient biopsychosocial factors perpetuating disability appear to have the best chance of returning disabled persons to a functional quality of life.
- See also *Fast Facts: Low Back Pain*.

Fibromyalgia

Fibromyalgia is characterized by:
- chronic widespread pain
- multiple tender points
- fatigue
- poor-quality sleep
- psychological distress and higher rates of comorbid mood disorder, in both patients and families.

The condition is more common in women, and its incidence appears to increase through middle age, after which it declines. The prevalence of fibromyalgia in the general population ranges from 0.5% to 5%, but it could be as high as 10% in women aged between 55 and 64 years. Symptoms may last for years, and relapses are common.

There is debate as to whether fibromyalgia constitutes a unique clinical entity or disease process because of the considerable overlap between patients with fibromyalgia and those with other unexplained syndromes such as irritable bowel syndrome, chronic fatigue syndrome and atypical chest pain, and because of the high association with mood disorder.

Pathophysiology. The pathophysiology of fibromyalgia remains uncertain. To date, the multidimensional (mechanical, thermal and electrical) hyperalgesia observed in patients with fibromyalgia has been explained in terms of a diffuse central sensitization leading to centrally generated symptoms and/or abnormal processing of normal sensory input. Brain-imaging studies support this explanation. Altered cytokine profiles may underlie peripheral or central sensitization.

The fatigue and sleep disturbances associated with this condition have been attributed to alterations in the hypothalamic–pituitary–adrenal (HPA) axis caused by hyperactivity of neurons that express corticotropin-releasing hormone. Cytokines have the capacity to disrupt the normal function of the HPA axis.

Diagnosis. Fibromyalgia is a clinical syndrome with no known confirmatory laboratory test. Clinical diagnosis is made on the basis of a history of widespread pain and pain triggered by digital palpation of at least 11 of 18 tender points (Figure 9.2). The pain tends to be diffuse, aching or burning, and is often described as 'head to toe'.

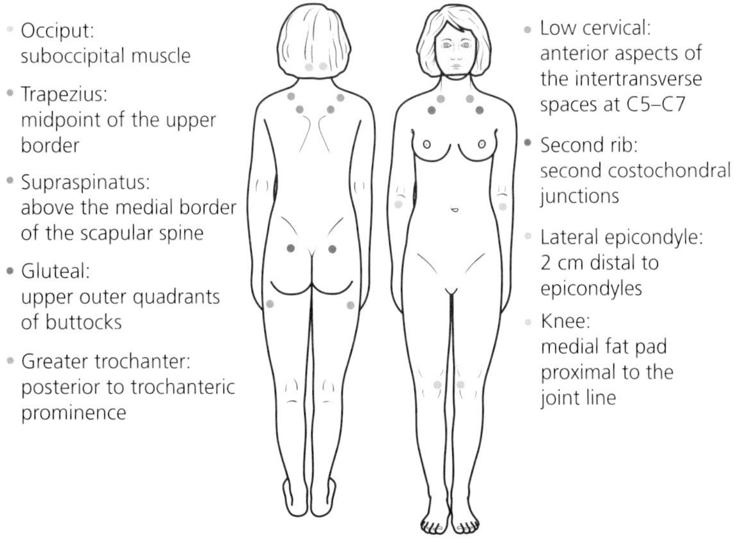

- Occiput:
  suboccipital muscle

- Trapezius:
  midpoint of the upper border

- Supraspinatus:
  above the medial border of the scapular spine

- Gluteal:
  upper outer quadrants of buttocks

- Greater trochanter:
  posterior to trochanteric prominence

- Low cervical:
  anterior aspects of the intertransverse spaces at C5–C7

- Second rib:
  second costochondral junctions

- Lateral epicondyle:
  2 cm distal to epicondyles

- Knee:
  medial fat pad proximal to the joint line

Figure 9.2 Tender points that indicate the presence of fibromyalgia.

Pharmacological management

NSAIDs. Paracetamol and NSAIDs are commonly used to relieve pain in patients with fibromyalgia. However, RCTs have found no clear benefit of NSAIDs over placebo for this condition, which is understandable given that there is no etiologic inflammatory process associated with fibromyalgia pain. When combined with antidepressants, NSAIDs may confer a slight incremental analgesic benefit. However, some authors argue that as there is no clear additional benefit, and given their potential toxicity, NSAID use is not cost-effective in the long term.

Antidepressants. A meta-analysis of RCTs has confirmed that the antidepressant classes of tricyclics and serotonin–norepinephrine-reuptake inhibitors (SNRIs) such as duloxetine and milnacipran relieve stiffness, reduce tenderness and improve sleep quality in fibromyalgia. On the other hand, evidence for the effectiveness of selective serotonin-reuptake inhibitors (SSRIs) is conflicting.

Muscle relaxants. RCTs show that cyclobenzaprine, a tricyclic marketed in the USA as a muscle relaxant, is effective for fibromyalgia pain.

Weak opioids. The SNRI properties of tramadol, in addition to its weak opioid agonist activity, suggest this as a candidate for moderate fibromyalgia pain. RCTs evaluating the efficacy of tramadol and paracetamol have found that the combination of these two drugs is superior to placebo for decreasing pain intensity in fibromyalgia. However, the follow-up period was short, and the potential for tolerance and dependence has not yet been elucidated (see pages 64–5).

Anticonvulsants. The gabapentinoid pregabalin has been shown to produce small-to-modest benefits in patients with fibromyalgia. The results of an RCT have suggested that pregabalin reduces pain, improves sleep and reduces fatigue in patients with fibromyalgia. Pregabalin provides pain relief in 1 in every 6 individuals, but minor adverse events also occur with the same prevalence.

Non-pharmacological treatment

Exercise. RCTs have demonstrated that aerobic exercise improves physical symptoms and anxiety scores. However, the minimal or optimal exercise regimen to produce such benefits has not yet been defined. The general approach is to combine a progressive exercise program with CBT and psychological support.

Acupuncture. There is conflicting evidence for the effectiveness of acupuncture for fibromyalgia. A systematic review of the literature could not account for the wide diversity of study results, though there is evidence of long-term benefits.

Education may include strategies for coping with symptoms, encouraging physical activity and discussion of biomedical knowledge with health providers. However, a systematic review of the efficacy of these types of program produced disappointing results as their benefits were not maintained at follow-up.

Prognosis. With appropriate treatment, mild-to-moderate fibromyalgia is not necessarily physically debilitating. The condition does not reduce life span.

Key points – fibromyalgia

- Fibromyalgia is characterized by chronic widespread pain, tender points, fatigue and poor sleep quality.
- Whether fibromyalgia constitutes a unique disease process is debated.
- Fibromyalgia is a clinical syndrome; there is no laboratory test that confirms the diagnosis.
- Exercise, tricyclic and serotonin–norepinephrine-reuptake inhibitor antidepressants, and cyclobenzaprine (with tricyclic antidepressant mechanism of action) are effective treatments.
- Pregabalin has small-to-modest analgesic efficacy.

Pain due to osteoporosis

Osteoporosis is a systemic skeletal condition characterized by decreased bone density and weakened bone structure that leads to an increased risk of bone fracture.

The most common primary forms of bone loss are postmenopausal and age-related osteoporosis. Osteoporosis may also be secondary to a wide variety of medical problems, including hypercortisolism, hyperthyroidism, and long-term use of corticosteroids, hyperparathyroidism, alcohol abuse and immobilization.

Approximately 25% of postmenopausal women have osteoporosis, and in people 60 years of age or older it is the most common risk factor for non-traumatic fractures. Osteoporosis produces chronic pain due to fractures. Vertebral fracture is the most frequent complication of osteoporosis (Figure 9.3) and is associated with high rates of chronic pain, functional decline, psychosocial dysfunction and early mortality.

Diagnosis. The earliest symptom of osteoporosis is often an episode of acute severe back pain caused by a vertebral compression fracture, or acute severe groin or thigh pain caused by a hip fracture. Diagnostic work-up should include a clinical history, physical examination, laboratory evaluation, bone densitometry and radiographic imaging. This work-up will generally allow the clinician to determine the cause of osteoporosis and to institute medical interventions to slow progression or even reverse the condition.

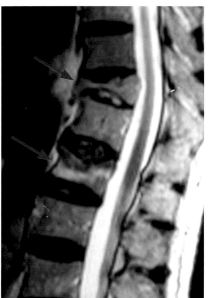

Figure 9.3 MRI scan showing two osteoporotic vertebral fractures in the thoracic region (red arrows). The lower fracture is a recent one.

General management. The choice of pain treatment should be tailored to the individual, as there is wide variation in the clinical presentation and the degree of physical disability associated with osteoporosis. For patients with acute or chronic pain, the treatment of pain and functional limitations should be the first priority.

Subsequent measures should include treatments aimed at maintaining bone mass to avoid new fractures, lifestyle re-education, physical therapy, physical fitness training, an appropriate course of rehabilitation to rebuild muscle mass and function, neurological and orthopedic evaluation and, for some patients, use of an orthosis.

Pharmacological management

NSAIDs are first-line treatment for mild-to-moderate pain secondary to a stable fracture. No trials have assessed the effect of NSAIDs on the healing of osteoporotic fractures. However, retrospective cohort studies have suggested that high doses of traditional NSAIDs could increase the likelihood of non-union after spinal fusion surgery. Conversely, RCTs that have evaluated bone healing after spinal fusion have provided no evidence that cyclooxygenase-2 (COX-2) inhibitors affect the rate of non-union at 1 year.

If pain persists, an opioid should be added. For any but the briefest of courses, opioid therapy should be approached as it is for any subacute-to-chronic illness. In this mostly elderly population, the approach to opioid therapy should include the initiation of a bowel regimen at the onset of therapy (see page 100), consideration of breakthrough medication as needed and controlled-release formulations.

When prescribing NSAIDs or opioids, the usual cautions with respect to comorbidity (e.g. with renal or pulmonary disease, respectively) should be kept in mind.

Calcitonin is a natural hormone that exerts antiresorptive properties by blocking osteoclastic activity. The value of calcitonin treatment for postmenopausal osteoporosis remains uncertain, particularly in the prevention of fractures. However, RCTs that have evaluated calcitonin administered after fractures indicate that, given subcutaneously or intranasally, it acts as an analgesic. Pain relief occurs within 1 week of starting calcitonin. Patients also seem to have earlier mobilization than those receiving a placebo.

The mechanism of calcitonin action is not yet known. It could be mediated through an effect on nociceptive transmission or on calcitonin-binding sites in areas of the brain. Further research is required to compare the efficacy of calcitonin with standard analgesics, as 1 in every 11 individuals given calcitonin stops taking it because of adverse events such as flushing, nausea and vomiting.

Epidural analgesia. In severe acute pain refractory to systemic medications, a short-term epidural catheter may aid mobilization in patients who would otherwise be bed-bound. The catheter tip is usually placed as close as possible to the fracture, and small doses of an opioid and local anesthetic are infused. Evidence for the effectiveness of this approach is only available from case reports.

Corticosteroid injection. Similar empirical results have shown that a single epidural injection of a corticosteroid provides symptomatic relief of inflammation adjoining a new vertebral fracture. Repeated injections, however, may enhance osteoporosis and so are relatively contraindicated.

Non-pharmacological treatment

Vertebroplasty has recently been introduced for treatment of patients with osteoporosis who have acute or chronic pain following vertebral fracture. The procedure involves the injection of bone cement into the fractured vertebral body in an attempt to stabilize fractured segments and reduce pain. Case series have suggested that the procedure is associated with substantial short-term pain relief and improvements in health-related quality of life (HRQoL) that seem to persist at 6 months. Other benefits include prevention of recurrent pain, reversal of height loss and spinal deformity, and improved level of function.

In general, 1–10% of patients experience short-term complications, mainly from the extravasation of cement. These problems include increased pain and damage from pressure on the spinal cord or nerve roots, infection, bleeding and pneumothorax.

Possible long-term complications include local acceleration of bone resorption caused by the treatment itself or by a foreign-body reaction at the cement–bone interface, and increased risk of fracture in treated or adjacent vertebrae through changes in mechanical forces. Vertebroplasty has recently been evaluated in an RCT – surprisingly, there was no long-term benefit.

Kyphoplasty (sometimes referred to as balloon-assisted vertebroplasty) has been evaluated only in case series. Before injecting the cement-like material, a balloon is inserted and gently inflated inside the fractured vertebrae. Substantial pain relief has been reported during short follow-up periods.

Kyphoplasty offers a theoretical advantage over vertebroplasty as the former is believed to provide better restoration of height and better reduction of spine deformity; however, it is more expensive. To date, no head-to-head trials have compared kyphoplasty with vertebroplasty.

Key points – pain due to osteoporosis

- Osteoporosis increases the risk of bone fracture, of which vertebral fracture is the most common.
- Non-steroidal anti-inflammatory drugs are the treatment of choice for mild-to-moderate pain secondary to a fracture, followed by opioid therapy for more severe pain.
- In case series, vertebroplasty is associated with substantial short-term pain relief and improvements in health-related quality of life that seem to persist at 6 months.
- See also *Fast Facts: Osteoporosis, 6th edn.*

Pain due to osteoarthritis

Osteoarthritis is a disease characterized by joint pain, distortion of joint architecture and impaired function due to articular cartilage degeneration and local inflammation. It is the most common form of arthritis and the most common cause of disability in older adults.

Osteoarthritis affects an estimated 20 million people or more in the USA and 4.5 million people in the UK. The condition is more prevalent with advancing age: people over 35 years of age have an

11% prevalence of hip osteoarthritis that increases to 36% in people over 85 years of age. Similarly, 10% of individuals over 55 years old have knee pain due to osteoarthritis; 25% of these individuals are severely disabled.

Osteoarthritis is one of the ten leading causes of disease burden in the developed world. Pain and physical limitations produced by osteoarthritis substantially affect HRQoL. Individuals with osteoarthritis have a lower HRQoL than individuals with gastrointestinal or cardiovascular conditions, or chronic respiratory diseases.

Pathophysiology. Although the causes of osteoarthritis are not completely understood, the enzymatic and mechanical breakdown of the cartilage matrix is key to the pathophysiology of the condition. Healthy cartilage is able to transmit force between the joints while maintaining almost friction-free limb movement. In osteoarthritis, these biomechanical properties are compromised; however, it is not clear whether the degeneration of cartilage precedes the onset of the disease or is a result of it.

The integrity of normal articular cartilage is maintained by a balance between anabolic and catabolic processes. This balance is disrupted in osteoarthritis. Cartilage degeneration correlates with age: senescent chondrocytes have decreased mitotic activity and are less responsive to anabolic growth factors, and thus synthesize smaller amounts of functional proteins. All of these changes lead to progressive cartilage damage and decreased capacity for regeneration.

In osteoarthritis, chondrocytes also produce an excess of nitric oxide and other inflammatory mediators such as eicosanoids and cytokines. The excessive nitric oxide produces cellular injury, inhibits cartilage synthesis and renders the chondrocyte susceptible to cytokine-induced apoptosis. In addition to promoting cartilage damage, these inflammatory phenomena predispose the patient to peripheral nerve sensitization with subsequent central sensitization and chronic pain.

Bone is also structurally abnormal in osteoarthritis. Periarticular bone has increased turnover, decreased bone mineral content and a reduced number of trabeculae, which affect its biomechanical integrity.

Diagnosis. Patients with osteoarthritis typically have morning stiffness and swelling of the involved joint (Figure 9.4), with pain that tends to worsen on weight-bearing or activity, but improves with rest.

Physical examination often reveals tenderness on palpation, bony enlargement, crepitus with movement and/or limitation of joint motion. Unlike in rheumatoid arthritis and other inflammatory arthritides, the inflammation in osteoarthritis, if obvious at all, is usually mild and localized to the affected joint.

(a)

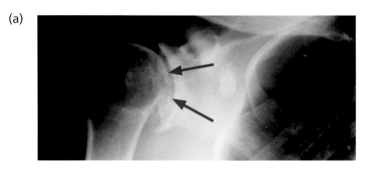

(b)

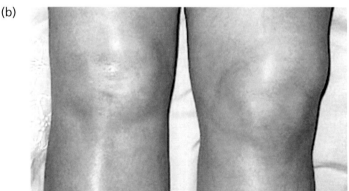

Figure 9.4 (a) Radiograph of a 65-year-old man with osteoarthritis of the shoulder. There is a marked decrease in the glenohumeral joint space (blue arrow), along with bony sclerosis (red arrow). (b) Osteoarthritis of both knees in a 67-year-old woman, with deformities and mild edema in the left knee.

General management. The goals of treatment for osteoarthritis are:
- pain relief
- prevention of complications such as muscle atrophy or deformities
- maintenance and/or improvement of functional status and HRQoL.

Treatment strategies consist of pharmacological and non-pharmacological modalities and invasive procedures.

Pharmacological management

NSAIDs. Meta-analyses have shown that NSAIDs are effective for pain relief in osteoarthritis: 59–82% of patients receiving NSAIDs report at least 50% pain relief. Paracetamol is less effective: only 20–40% of patients who receive paracetamol report pain relief of 50% or more.

Conventional NSAIDs inhibit both of the COX isoforms, COX-1 and COX-2, but COX-2 inhibitors are much more selective against the COX-2 isoform. The COX-1 isoform is produced constitutively (i.e. always produced), and it is present mainly in the gastric mucosa. COX-2 is inducible and is responsible for the enhanced formation of prostaglandins during inflammation.

Multiple RCTs have confirmed the effectiveness of COX-2 inhibitors for osteoarthritis. The major clinical interest of these selective COX-2 inhibitors has been the lower incidence of gastrointestinal bleeding than that associated with traditional NSAIDs; however, this benefit is not always present, decreases over time and falls with the concomitant use of ASA (for cardiovascular protection).

A comprehensive study of the cost-effectiveness of COX-2 inhibitors and traditional NSAIDs has found that money saved from the risk reduction of gastrointestinal adverse effects associated with COX-2 inhibitors does not offset the higher costs of these drugs during management of average-risk patients with chronic arthritis.

In addition, growing concern regarding an increase in cardiovascular events in patients receiving COX-2 inhibitors led to the withdrawal of rofecoxib and valdecoxib from the market in the USA and re-evaluation of their status in Europe. Following a thorough review in the USA and Australia, celecoxib remains on the market because of its favorable gastrointestinal safety profile.

While the efficacy and safety of NSAIDs and COX-2 inhibitors for long-term use are being re-evaluated, it seems most prudent to employ long-established NSAIDs for pain relief after careful patient selection and with ongoing monitoring. Patients receiving long-term treatment with either NSAIDs or COX-2 inhibitors should be informed that all drugs in these classes (except for ASA) carry cardiovascular risks with chronic use.

Combination therapy. The combination of NSAIDs and weak opioids (e.g. paracetamol with codeine or tramadol) seems to provide slightly greater analgesia than paracetamol alone in patients with osteoarthritis, as double-blind RCTs have shown.

Strong opioids. Given alone or in combination with NSAIDs or paracetamol, strong opioids are effective for chronic arthritis pain. Controlled-release preparations (oral or transdermal) of agents such as morphine, oxycodone and fentanyl, as well as of the partial opioid agonist buprenorphine, are suitable for long-term use.

Glucosamine is a widely used therapy, but its effectiveness is unproven.

Tricyclic antidepressants. Meta-analyses of RCTs have confirmed that tricyclic antidepressants are effective for the treatment of osteoarthritic pain.

Capsaicin. A systematic review of published RCTs found that capsaicin decreased osteoarthritic pain (see page 68 for a general description of capsaicin).

Intra-articular therapy. When patients do not respond to a program of non-pharmacological therapy (see below) and analgesics, intra-articular injections of sodium hyaluronate or corticosteroids produce symptomatic benefit that may last for as long as 6 months. However, limited data are available on the effectiveness of multiple courses of intra-articular therapy.

Surgery. Total joint replacement, such as total hip and total knee arthroplasties, are extremely effective in improving dimensions of HRQoL. Logic and evidence indicate that the timing of surgery should be individualized on the basis of response to less invasive options and with orthopedic specialist consultation.

Indications for joint replacement include radiographic evidence of joint damage and/or moderate-to-severe persistent pain or disability that are not substantially relieved by an extended course of non-surgical management.

Non-pharmacological treatment

Exercise and weight loss. Exercise reduces pain and disability in patients with osteoarthritis of the hip or knee. These findings are supported by systematic reviews of the literature and a meta-analysis of RCTs on the effect of exercise on osteoarthritic pain.

Consistently, RCTs show that overweight patients with hip or knee osteoarthritis who lose weight have improved symptoms and function.

Education. A systematic review of published RCTs and non-randomized trials has suggested a beneficial effect of educational programs such as relaxation training, biofeedback, problem-solving strategies, social support or stress reduction for patients with osteoarthritis. These programs have been shown to reduce joint pain and the frequency of arthritis-related physician visits, increase physical activity and improve quality of life.

Acupuncture. The role of acupuncture for the treatment of osteoarthritis is not clear. RCTs have shown that acupuncture is not superior to sham-needling in reducing osteoarthritic pain. This equivalence implies that sham-needling has similar specific effects as acupuncture or that both methods produce substantial non-specific effects.

In the future, efforts to prevent the development or progression of osteoarthritis will probably include strategies that delay the onset of chondrocyte senescence or that replace senescent cells. These objectives can be met by disease-modifying drugs aimed at inhibiting the breakdown of cartilage or at stimulating repair activity by chondrocytes.

Key points – pain due to osteoarthritis

- Osteoarthritis is characterized by joint pain with loss of joint architecture and function due to articular cartilage degeneration and local inflammation.
- Pain and limitation of physical function substantially affect health-related quality of life (HRQoL).
- The goal of treatment is to relieve pain, prevent complications and maintain and/or improve functional status and HRQoL.
- Exercise and weight loss are beneficial.
- Non-steroidal anti-inflammatory drugs (NSAIDs) are effective for pain relief.
- Ongoing concerns regarding the safety and cost-effectiveness of chronic therapy with cyclooxygenase (COX)-2 inhibitors has led to worldwide caution over their use.
- Patients treated long term with NSAIDs or COX-2 inhibitors should be informed that all drugs in these classes (except ASA) carry cardiovascular risks with chronic use.
- Total joint arthroplasties are effective for improving HRQoL.
- See also *Fast Facts: Osteoarthritis.*

Pain due to rheumatoid arthritis

Rheumatoid arthritis is a chronic systemic autoimmune disorder characterized by joint pain and inflammation that may progress to joint destruction. Rheumatoid arthritis is the most common inflammatory arthritis and a major cause of disability; 1–2% of the world's population is affected by the condition.

Pathophysiology. A multistage theory that integrates various genetic hypotheses has been postulated. Some believe that rheumatoid arthritis originates from a bacterial or viral infection. Bacterial and viral antigenic particles have been detected in synovial tissue, and could be responsible for the initial activation of the inflammation. B cell activation and generation of autoantibodies directed to the Fc ('fragment that crystallizes') portion of human immunoglobulin G

131

class molecules ('rheumatoid factors') could also be responsible for activation of innate immunity. The production of cytokines such as tumor necrosis factor-α and interleukin-1 by macrophages and fibroblasts in the joint, and the local expression of adhesion molecules following immune activation, promote the ingress of immune cells and the accumulation of T cells and B cells in the inflamed synovium. Cytokines and locally expressed degradative enzymes such as metalloproteinases digest the cartilage matrix and destroy articular and bone structures, resulting in pain.

Diagnosis of rheumatoid arthritis requires the presence of four or more of the criteria shown in Table 9.3. Subluxation of the atlantoaxial or cricoarytenoid joints may not be apparent, but patients with cervical spine instability are at risk of impingement of the spinal cord during routine procedures such as endotracheal intubation, and should therefore undergo neurological evaluation before any surgical intervention. Hoarseness or pain on talking should alert the clinician to possible problems with the cricoarytenoid joint.

TABLE 9.3

Criteria for diagnosis of rheumatoid arthritis

Diagnose if ≥ 4 of the following features are present

- Morning stiffness in and around joints for ≥ 1 hour before maximal improvement*
- Soft tissue swelling of ≥ 3 joint areas*
- Swelling of the proximal interphalangeal, metacarpophalangeal or wrist joints*
- Symmetric swelling*
- Subcutaneous rheumatoid nodules
- Circulating rheumatoid factor
- Radiographic erosions and/or periarticular osteopenia in hand and/or wrist joints (Figure 9.5)

*Must have been present for at least 6 weeks.

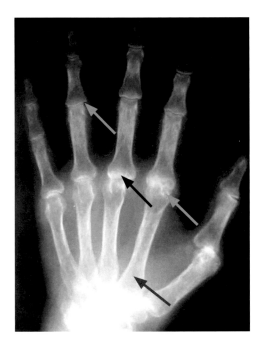

Figure 9.5 Radiograph of the hand of a 48-year-old woman with rheumatoid arthritis, showing diffuse osteopenia (red arrow), decreased interphalangeal joint spaces without sclerosis (black arrow) and subchondral cysts (blue arrows). Similar changes are observed in the carpal joints.

Pharmacological management

NSAIDs. Traditionally, pharmacotherapy for rheumatoid arthritis follows a 'pyramid model' in which the first level of treatment is NSAID therapy. Meta-analysis of RCTs has confirmed that NSAIDs are effective in decreasing pain and the number of tender joints, and improving function in rheumatoid arthritis.

COX-2 inhibitors and traditional NSAIDs have similar analgesic efficacy. However, COX-2 inhibitors should not be considered as first-line treatment (see pages 128–9 for the supporting arguments).

NSAID–opioid combinations. The combination of NSAIDs and weak opioids is commonly used to produce greater analgesia than can be achieved by each individual drug.

Slow-acting antirheumatic drugs (SAARDs) are used to replace or supplement NSAIDs when the latter do not provide adequate pain control. SAARDs are distinguished from NSAIDs primarily by their assumed disease-modifying potential and delayed onset of action. Agents falling within this therapeutic class include hydroxychloroquine, gold, D-penicillamine, methotrexate, azathioprine

133

and sulfasalazine. In much of the literature this class is also termed 'disease-modifying antirheumatic drugs' (DMARDs).

Systematic reviews of RCTs that have evaluated SAARDs have confirmed their effectiveness in reducing pain intensity and decreasing the number of painful and swollen joints. However, their use is associated with a high discontinuation rate due to adverse events, especially for azathioprine and cyclophosphamide.

Oral corticosteroids decrease joint tenderness and pain, and improve grip strength with an efficacy nearly equivalent to second-line agents previously examined in meta-analyses. The morbidity associated with chronic corticosteroid use mandates great caution in their use.

One RCT has suggested that SAARDs produce their greatest benefit when introduced early in the course of the disease.

Biological response modifiers (BRMs) are a third line of treatment based on pathogenic mechanisms. BRMs are DMARD treatments aimed at blocking the specific biological effects of inflammatory cytokines, tumor necrosis factor and other modulators of inflammation.

RCTs have indicated that BRMs are more efficacious than traditional agents because, in addition to addressing symptoms, they attenuate synovial inflammation, halt the progression of joint damage and joint destruction, and reduce disease activity in patients with long-standing rheumatoid arthritis. One-quarter of individuals treated with BRMs obtain substantial pain relief. However, the side effects may be serious, and include severe infection, increased risk of tuberculosis, lymphomas and demyelinating disease.

Tricyclic antidepressants. RCTs have consistently shown that antidepressants are efficacious for pain associated with rheumatoid arthritis and therefore should be an early part of the treatment armamentarium.

Non-pharmacological treatment

Education. A systematic review of the literature has concluded that patient education is effective in reducing pain and improving function in rheumatoid arthritis. The programs reviewed included relaxation training, biofeedback, problem-solving strategies, social support and stress reduction. Comparing its relative effectiveness with that of modalities such as NSAIDs, education gives 20–30% greater benefit overall; education is also 40% better than NSAIDs at improving functional ability and 60–80% better at reducing tender joint counts.

A systematic review of RCTs that have evaluated the effect of relaxation, biofeedback and cognitive behavioral therapies suggests that each of these therapies is an effective adjunctive treatment.

Occupational therapy improves functional ability in patients with rheumatoid arthritis, according to the results of a systematic review of RCTs.

Exercise. A meta-analysis of RCTs has shown that exercise in patients with well-controlled disease increases aerobic capacity, joint mobility and muscle strength.

Acupuncture has not been found to be of use for the treatment of pain associated with rheumatoid arthritis.

Key points – pain due to rheumatoid arthritis

- Rheumatoid arthritis is a chronic systemic autoimmune disorder characterized by joint inflammation, joint destruction and pain.
- Education, occupational therapy, exercise, relaxation, biofeedback and cognitive behavioral therapies are effective interventions.
- Pharmacological treatment follows a pyramidal model: it begins with NSAIDs, is followed by slow-acting antirheumatic drugs and ends with biological response modifiers.
- Joint replacement is appropriate for the restoration of function in joints deformed by advanced rheumatoid arthritis, but intubation for anesthesia must be approached cautiously in light of potential unappreciated cricoarytenoid or atlantoaxial joint subluxation.
- See also *Fast Facts: Rheumatoid Arthritis, 2nd edn.*

Key references

Atlas SJ, Keller RB, Chang Y et al. Surgical and nonsurgical management of sciatica secondary to a lumbar disc herniation: five-year outcomes from the Maine Lumbar Spine Study. *Spine (Phila Pa 1976)* 2001;26:1179–87.

Cepeda MS, Camargo F, Zea C, Valencia L. Tramadol for osteoarthritis. *Cochrane Database Syst Rev* 2006, issue 3. CD005522. www.thecochranelibrary.com

Deyo RA. Diagnostic evaluation of LBP: reaching a specific diagnosis is often impossible. *Arch Intern Med* 2002;162:1444–7; discussion 47–8.

Firestein GS. Evolving concepts of rheumatoid arthritis. *Nature* 2003;423:356–61.

Fishbain D. Evidence-based data on pain relief with antidepressants. *Ann Med* 2000;32:305–16.

Hayden JA, van Tulder MW, Tomlinson G. Systematic review: strategies for using exercise therapy to improve outcomes in chronic low back pain. *Ann Intern Med* 2005;142:776–85.

Jarvik JG, Hollingworth W, Martin B et al. Rapid magnetic resonance imaging vs radiographs for patients with low back pain: a randomized controlled trial. *JAMA* 2003;289:2810–18.

Linton SJ, van Tulder MW. Preventive interventions for back and neck pain problems: what is the evidence? *Spine (Phila Pa 1976)* 2001;26:778–87.

Manheimer E, White A, Berman B et al. Meta-analysis: acupuncture for low back pain. *Ann Intern Med* 2005;142:651–63.

Messier SP, Loeser RF, Miller GD et al. Exercise and dietary weight loss in overweight and obese older adults with knee osteoarthritis: the Arthritis, Diet, and Activity Promotion Trial. *Arthritis Rheum* 2004;50:1501–10.

Peul WC, van Houwelingen HC, van den Hout WB et al. Surgery versus prolonged conservative treatment for sciatica. *N Engl J Med* 2007;356:2245–56.

Salerno SM, Browning R, Jackson JL. The effect of antidepressant treatment on chronic back pain: a meta-analysis. *Arch Intern Med* 2002;162:19–24.

Spiegel BM, Targownik L, Dulai GS, Gralnek IM. The cost-effectiveness of cyclooxygenase-2 selective inhibitors in the management of chronic arthritis. *Ann Intern Med* 2003;138:795–806.

In the past, viscera were considered insensitive to pain. It is now clear that visceral pain results from the activation of sensory afferent nerves that innervate internal organs such as the stomach, kidney, gallbladder, urinary bladder, intestines or pancreas. Disorders that could trigger visceral pain include distension from impaction, tumors, ischemia, inflammation and traction on the mesentery. There are a variety of pain syndromes thought to be maintained by the persistent activation of visceral nociceptive fibers. However, there is a common pathophysiology and symptomatic management approach to all of these syndromes.

Pathophysiology

Nociceptive input from the body surface travels along somatic nerves that enter spinal roots, accounting for the clear dermatomal organization of somatic pain sensations. Nociceptive information from internal organs, which are exclusively innervated by Aδ and unmyelinated C fibers, travels via more diffusely organized sympathetic and parasympathetic afferent pathways that enter the spinal cord at the thoracic and lumbar levels. In addition, visceral afferent fibers contain a greater percentage of neuroexcitatory transmitters such as substance P than do somatic afferent fibers. These differences between somatic and visceral innervation explain why sensations arising from visceral stimulation are generally more diffuse, more difficult to localize and more unpleasant than somatic sensations, and also why they are referred to poorly localized regions of the body surface. Visceral sensations are often accompanied by autonomic reflexes and symptoms such as nausea, sweating and malaise.

Three physiological classes of nociceptive viscerosensory receptors exist:
- high-threshold, which respond only to noxious mechanical stimuli
- wide-dynamic-range, which encode a wide range of innocuous and noxious stimuli
- silent, which are activated by inflammation.

High-threshold receptors exclusively innervate organs from which pain is the only conscious sensation (e.g. ureter, kidney, lungs, heart), but there are relatively few of this receptor type in organs that provide both innocuous and noxious sensations (e.g. colon, stomach, bladder).

The etiology of persistent visceral pain is still not certain. However, it is clear that visceral pain is not always linked to injury. It is believed that persistent activation of visceral fibers leads to central sensitization and to visceral hyperalgesia and that, just as for hyperalgesia from chronic somatic pain, excessive activity of N-methyl D-aspartate (NMDA) receptors is involved in this process. Autoimmune responses and inflammation could trigger the persistent activation of visceral afferent fibers. The possibility that visceral nerve injury may give rise to persistent visceral neuropathic pain is embodied in the term 'complex regional pain syndrome' (see Chapter 4).

Symptomatic management

Treatment of visceral chronic pain syndromes is aimed at symptomatic pain management. Today, visceral pain management focuses on both pharmacological and interventional techniques. Combinations of non-steroidal anti-inflammatory drugs (NSAIDs), adjuvant medications and opioids, in that sequence, form the mainstay of therapy. When pharmacological therapies prove ineffective or are limited by side effects, regional anesthesia techniques, neurostimulation (peripheral or spinal cord) or neurosurgical techniques are considered. However, the effectiveness of these last therapies has not been evaluated rigorously, and therefore they should only be used as a last resort.

In addition, there are specific treatment modalities that are used for the treatment of specific pain syndromes.

For illustrative purposes, this chapter discusses:
- irritable bowel syndrome (IBS)
- interstitial cystitis
- male chronic pelvic pain syndrome
- endometriosis.

Irritable bowel syndrome

As much as 20% of the adult population exhibits symptoms of IBS. This functional disorder is characterized by abdominal pain, cramping, bloating, constipation and diarrhea. It occurs more often in women than in men, and it begins before the age of 35 in half of those afflicted. Most people can control their symptoms with diet, stress management and medications, but for some it can be disabling, preventing them from working, attending social events or traveling even short distances.

Diagnosis. Because IBS has no pathognomonic physical signs, its diagnosis usually requires exclusion of structural pathology with imaging or more invasive testing. It cannot be diagnosed solely from the patient's medical history. Inclusion criteria for diagnosis are shown in Table 10.1.

Treatment. Mild symptoms of IBS usually respond to stress management and changes in diet and lifestyle. If symptoms persist despite judicious use of laxatives for constipation, antidiarrheal agents or antispasmodics, tricyclic antidepressants may relieve pain and diarrhea, as one of their side effects is constipation.

As the autonomic nervous system and its enteric compartment play an important role in regulating motility and visceral perception, neurotransmitters (particularly serotonin) are targets for novel pharmacotherapeutic agents for this syndrome. Specific medications for IBS include tegaserod, a partially selective serotonin agonist (not available in the UK).

TABLE 10.1

Criteria for the diagnosis of irritable bowel syndrome

- Abdominal pain*
- Diarrhea or constipation lasting at least 12 weeks*

Plus ≥ 2 of:

- change in the frequency of bowel movements
- change in the consistency of stool
- straining
- urgency
- a feeling of incomplete bowel movement or bloating
- mucus in the stool

*Do not have to occur consecutively.
See also *Fast Facts: Irritable Bowel Syndrome*.

Interstitial cystitis

Interstitial cystitis is a heterogeneous chronic pain syndrome that most commonly affects women (90%). Symptoms include pain on bladder filling, pelvic pain and urinary urgency and frequency. The symptoms are often exacerbated by ovulation and during periods of stress.

Diagnosis. In the absence of practical clinical criteria for the diagnosis of interstitial cystitis, the US National Institute of Diabetes and Digestive and Kidney Diseases of the National Institutes of Health developed criteria for research purposes. These criteria were never meant to be a gold standard for diagnosis, but they are often used as such. To be diagnosed with interstitial cystitis for research purposes, patients must have glomerulations or Hunner's ulcer on cystoscopic examination, and either bladder pain or urinary urgency in the absence of other diseases that could cause the symptoms.

Treatment. Hydrodistention of the bladder, intravesical instillation therapy and transurethral resection of diseased bladder tissue have been used to treat interstitial cystitis. However, the effectiveness of these therapies has not been evaluated rigorously. Commonly used non-surgical management strategies include paying careful attention to diet to avoid acidic foods that might acidify the urine. Sacral nerve stimulation has been reported to be effective for extremely intractable pain, however no controlled studies are available.

Male chronic pelvic pain syndrome

The diagnosis of male chronic pelvic pain syndrome is made in men who complain of chronic pelvic pain but who have an unrevealing examination and work-up. Interstitial cystitis (see above) and male chronic pelvic pain syndrome may be the same syndrome.

Endometriosis

Endometriosis is a common gynecologic condition that produces cyclical pain. Women complain of severe dysmenorrhea, focal pelvic tenderness and dyspareunia. The pain arises because of the dissemination of endometrium to ectopic sites during retrograde menstruation or surgery, and the subsequent establishment of deposits of ectopic endometrial tissue.

In many women, endometriosis is a self-limiting disease; however, in others the biological behavior is much more unpredictable.

Diagnosis is made by laparoscopy.

Treatment of endometriosis includes therapies such as medroxyprogesterone acetate, danazol, nafarelin and gonadotropin-releasing hormone analogs. Medical therapy after surgical treatment reduces pain substantially, but trials have shown that there is no difference postoperatively at 6 months whether or not medical therapy is used. Although the efficacy of a variety of treatments has been demonstrated in randomized controlled trials, only 40–70% of women with severe cases of endometriosis become pain free.

Key points – visceral pain

- Visceral pain results from activation of sensory afferent nerves that innervate the stomach, kidney, gallbladder, urinary bladder, intestines, pancreas and other visceral organs.
- Sensations arising from visceral stimulation are generally more diffuse, more difficult to localize and more unpleasant than those associated with somatic pain.
- Visceral pain is more likely than somatic pain to be associated with autonomic signs such as pallor and sweating, or symptoms such as nausea.
- Pain syndromes such as male chronic pelvic pain syndrome, interstitial cystitis, endometriosis and irritable bowel syndrome are thought to be maintained by the persistent activation of visceral fibers, and central sensitization.
- Management includes identifying and avoiding factors that aggravate the underlying condition and individual clinical trials of medication. Neuromodulatory techniques have been reported as helpful in selected cases.

Key references

Al-Chaer ED, Traub RJ. Biological basis of visceral pain: recent developments. *Pain* 2002;96:221–5.

Batstone GR, Doble A. Chronic prostatitis. *Curr Opin Urol* 2003;13:23–9.

Giamberardino MA. Visceral pain. *Pain: Clinical Updates* 2005;XIII. www.iasp-pain.org

Howard FM. An evidence-based medicine approach to the treatment of endometriosis-associated chronic pelvic pain: placebo-controlled studies. *J Am Assoc Gynecol Laparosc* 2000;7:477–88.

Kream RM, Carr DB. Interstitial cystitis: a complex visceral pain syndrome. *Pain Forum* 1999;8:139–45.

Peeker R, Fall M. Treatment guidelines for classic and non-ulcer interstitial cystitis. *Int Urogynecol J Pelvic Floor Dysfunct* 2000;11:23–32.

Prentice A, Deary AJ, Goldbeck-Wood S et al. Gonadotrophin-releasing hormone analogues for pain associated with endometriosis. *Cochrane Database Syst Rev* 2000, issue 2. CD000346. www.thecochranelibrary.com

Strigo IA, Bushnell MC, Boivin M, Duncan GH. Psychophysical analysis of visceral and cutaneous pain in human subjects. *Pain* 2002;97:235–46.

Wesselmann U, Czakanski PP. Pelvic pain: a chronic visceral pain syndrome. *Curr Pain Headache Rep* 2001;5:13–9.

Headache is a common complaint in the general population and one of the most common reasons people seek care from primary care providers.

Classification

Acute headache. The immediate, important first step in assessing a new headache is determining whether the headache is a serious, potentially life-threatening, medical event requiring emergency evaluation and management. All the possibilities highlighted in Table 11.1 must be entertained and discarded before considering the headache to be caused by a chronic headache condition. Brain imaging, including neurovascular studies, may be needed as well as

TABLE 11.1

Examples of circumstances requiring emergency evaluation and management

- Acute severe head pain with neurological symptoms in an adult with no prior history of headache may indicate a cerebral vascular accident, including bleeding aneurysm
- Headache and severe eye pain suggests possible acute glaucoma
- Co-occurrence of fever associated with pneumonia or other infection with stiff neck and other neurological signs may indicate meningitis or encephalitis
- Past history of cancer suggests the possibility of intracerebral tumor
- Recent head trauma or rapid acceleration/deceleration injury suggests the possibility of intracranial bleed
- History of head/neck trauma (or diagnostic lumbar puncture) followed by severe generalized headache markedly increased by upright postures suggests tear of dura or dural cuff causing leak of cerebrospinal fluid (CSF) and low CSF pressure

cerebrospinal fluid (CSF) pressure measurement and analysis and further evaluation by a neurologist.

Chronic headache

Assessment. As with all chronic pain, headache must be assessed systematically and classified according to its likely origin as well as its temporal pattern, aggravating and ameliorating factors and perpetuating factors and comorbidities. The headache diagnoses in Table 11.2 should be considered.

History. The history should note, as for any other pain, a general medical history, including a detailed pain history (Table 11.3). It is important to note whether the headache corresponds to any cycles

TABLE 11.2

Possible diagnoses for chronic headache

- Migraine: usually unilateral throbbing and episodic; often (~ 25%) preceded by aura; associated with sensory phobia to light, noise and movement

- Tension-type: usually band-like pain that is generally steady; often starts in occipital region

- Cluster: very intense and disabling; lasts for days to weeks at a time

- Sinus: with facial frontal pain, often associated with fever or allergies

- Occipital neuralgia and cervicogenic headache associated with cervical spine pathology

- Traumatic brain injury: can have multiple presentations in the context of a history of motor vehicle accidents, head trauma from falls or sports, or exposure to blast waves

- Mass lesion: from primary or secondary tumor, abscess or chronic subdural hematoma

- Transform headache: caused by frequent regular use of short-acting analgesics of any class (medication 'rebound' effects)

- Trigeminal neuralgia may sometimes present as headache (see Chapter 3) (menstruation, weekends, circadian) or particular exposures (fumes, smoke, foods, etc).

As emotional factors often trigger tension or migraine headache, psychosocial assessment for the relationship of stressful events to headache onset and extant stressors or psychiatric comorbidities will be important for risk management and treatment planning. Diagnostic testing, particularly brain imaging, may be appropriate.

Pathophysiology and associated signs and symptoms

Recent literature has tended to blur what were once thought to be clear distinctions between headaches without a clear anatomic generator, such as tension headache compared with migraine headache. However, it is useful to consider migraine headache and tension headache differently for therapeutic reasons.

Migraine headache is now thought to be a condition in which there is cortical neuronal hyperexcitability and/or brainstem dysfunction which activates peripheral nociceptors of the trigeminal neurovascular system. An increase in excitatory neurotransmitters such as glutamate and reduced intracortical inhibition are associated with meningeal inflammation and peripheral sensitization leading to dilation of cerebral vessels and pain. Further activation of the trigeminal nucleus leads to the characteristic signs of central sensitization usually associated with the clinical picture of full-blown migraine, during which almost any sensory stimulus will worsen the headache. These signs and symptoms include allodynia over the face and head, photophobia and sensitivity to noise or movement, causing patients to want to lie down in a dark, completely quiet room until the headache passes. There appears to be a genetic predisposition to migraine in some patients.

Tension headache, thought to be due to myofascial pain in the muscles of the head and neck, may be activated by stress and postural factors, or by neural stimuli from an old injury and/or cervical spine disease. These headaches can themselves activate a migraine headache in some patients.

TABLE 11.3

Diagnostic indicators that can be obtained from a careful history

Headache type	Location	Precipitants
Tension	Often bilateral Starts in occipital region	Stress, postural factors, injury, cervical spine disease
Migraine	Usually unilateral Temples	Triggers in order of decreasing frequency: • stress (~ 75%) • menstruation • not eating • weather changes • sleep loss • odors • neck pain • bright lights • alcohol • smoke • food • heat • exercise (~ 20%)
Cluster	Usually unilateral (side may change in 15%)	Seasonal for some
Chronic paroxysmal hemicrania (CPH)	Ocular, frontal, temporal and adjacent areas	Sometimes neck movement
Sinus	Facial	Upper respiratory tract infection, allergies
Transform (rebound)		Regular, frequent dosing of short-acting medication
Occipital neuralgia	Occipital region, often starting in neck	Position of neck
Myofascial	Neck, occipital region	Position, spine pathology
Traumatic brain injury	Variable	History of trauma, sports, concussion

Pattern/progression	Duration	Frequency
Progressing to band-like headache	Hours, days (rarely)	Episodic
68% have prodrome of nausea, vomiting, visual or mood symptoms Progresses to throbbing headache that is usually unilateral and often disabling, with sensory sensitization	Hours, sometimes days	Episodic
Lacrimation, nasal stuffiness, photophobia	Several days	Once or several times yearly
Modified 'cluster pattern' Complete relief with indometacin (indomethacin)		Episodic
Sometimes fever, tender over sinuses		Episodic
	Chronic, daily	Chronic, daily
Can progress to migraine-type headache	Variable	Variable
	Variable	Variable
Can be refractory to treatment	Variable, can be constant	Variable, can be daily with migraine-type flares

Transform headache, often called rebound headache, is caused when the pain-suppressing effects of a short-acting sedative, anxiolytic and/ or analgesic wear off so that the manifestations of the sensitized state of the central nervous system (CNS) resumes. Hence caution against the regular, daily or almost daily use of these drugs for headache control is advised.

Sinus headache is caused by allergy- or infection-induced sinus inflammation with subsequent blockage and increased pressure.

Psychological processes. Stress is the most common trigger of both migraine (~75%) and tension headache, and like all persistent or recurrent pain, the headaches themselves and their effects on function and quality of life can be stressful to patients, their families and their associates.

Physical examination

While many common headaches can be diagnosed by history alone, to rule out dangerous causes, physical examination of the head and neck and cranial nerves as well as physiological parameters such as vital signs (e.g. fever) and mental status (with particular attention being paid to neurological function) is necessary. For example, palpation over the occipital nerve can precipitate the pain of occipital neuralgia and trigger points in the neck and trapezius can radiate rostrally causing headache. Palpation of a very prominent and sensitive superficial temporal artery can point to a possible diagnosis of temporal arteritis; this is a crucial diagnosis because if left untreated blindness is a likely complication.

Signs and symptoms of cervical spine pathology, such as tenderness over upper cervical facet joints may point to a need for imaging or cervical spine and possible diagnostic medial branch blocks; this could lead to a diagnosis of 'cervicogenic headache'. As emotional factors often trigger tension or migraine headache, psychosocial assessment for stressors or psychiatric comorbidity is important.

Diagnostic testing, particularly brain imaging, may be appropriate to rule out intracerebral causes.

Diagnostic tests

For most chronic headaches, diagnostic tests are unnecessary except when a 'red flag' on history or physical examination indicates concern for intracerebral mass and the need for imaging, or history and physical examination indicate a need for spinal evaluation and related imaging. In occipital neuralgia, sometimes neural blockade of the occipital nerves can help with diagnosis. Administration of indometacin (indomethacin) results in complete relief of chronic paroxysmal hemicrania (CPH) and this effect continues with long-term treatment. Cluster headache diagnosis may be aided by the autonomic features and at least partial response to inhaled oxygen.

Treatment

Migraine. The treatment approach for migraine is best conceptualized as longitudinal chronic disease management, in three parts: preventive measures, abortive treatment and symptom management. This approach is based on understanding the phenomenological pattern of each individual's headache, as in Figure 11.1.

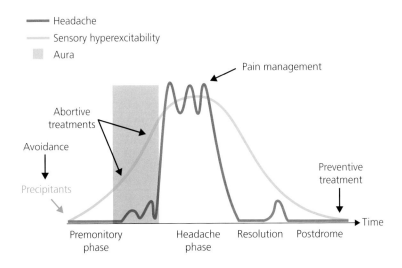

Figure 11.1 The natural course of a typical migraine attack. Adapted with permission from Linde M. *Acta Neurol Scand* 2006;114:71–83.

First, preventive treatments aim to reduce the frequency, severity and duration of attacks and include daily use of medications such as antidepressants, anticonvulsants, alpha$_2$ agonists, and beta-blockers (Table 11.4).

Second, once prodromal or actual migraine symptoms occur, a stepped-care approach should be taken (Table 11.5). It is important to avoid frequent regular dosing (more than twice weekly) of short-acting analgesics or sedatives such as compounds containing butalbital (a short-acting barbiturate often compounded with non-steroidal anti-inflammatory drugs [NSAIDs] or paracetamol [acetaminophen]), to reduce the incidence of transform (rebound) daily headaches.

Psychotherapies, such as support/directive and cognitive behavioral therapies (CBT), may help patients manage a complex interaction of factors that perpetuate headache.

Botulinum toxin injections have been reported to be successful in some case series, but the clinical trials are equivocal; a trial should be reserved for treatment-resistant patients.

TABLE 11.4

Preventive treatments for migraine headaches

Antidepressants

- SSRIs (e.g. sertraline, fluoxetine, citalopram)
- SNRIs (e.g. duloxetine, venlafaxine, milnacipran)
- Tricyclic antidepressants (e.g. amitriptyline)

Anticonvulsants

- Valproate
- Topiramate
- Gabapentin
- Pregabalin

Beta-blockers

- Propanolol

Others

- Verapamil

SNRI, serotonin–norepinephrine reuptake inhibitor; SSRI, selective serotonin-reuptake inhibitor.

TABLE 11.5

Stepped-care approach to adopt on occurrence of prodromal or actual migraine symptoms

- **Initial treatment:** attempt to abort progression to full-blown migraine by removing triggers, by relaxation and by oral NSAIDs
- **Next:** if initial treatment is not successful, oral or intramuscular or nasal triptans, which have high efficacy and are generally well tolerated, are indicated; several should be tried until the most effective abortive treatment is found
- **If migraine persists:** rescue doses of analgesics and sedatives such as short-acting opioids and benzodiazepines can be used. Inducing sleep often terminates the attack

NSAID, non-steroidal anti-inflammatory drug.

For intractable migraine and occipital neuralgia a form of neuromodulation may be trialed in the form of temporary insertion of suboccipital electrodes; about 50% of such patients proceed to permanent implantation of electrodes and pulse generator.

Tension headache. Management of episodic tension-type headaches starts with understanding the precipitants of the headaches. This is best accomplished by a headache diary in which the patient records all headaches and their contexts, either in a small notebook, on headache diary sheets or in a personal digital assistant (PDA). Once precipitants are identified, intervention strategies should proceed as follows.

- For stress-induced headache, a stress management program, usually delivered in CBT, that trains the patient to avoid and/or manage precipitating stressors and to relax and stretch at onset of headache.
- For positional headache, such as that activated by poor ergonomics at a computer terminal, positional and seating changes, stretching routines and icing can be helpful.

On onset of headache, modulation techniques are initiated, such as stretching and icing, and relaxation techniques. Usually analgesics such as NSAIDs or paracetamol suffice, although other medications such as tramadol may be tried in more severe forms. The medical custom in some countries, such as the USA, includes use of pills, combining a barbiturate, butalbital, and caffeine with paracetamol or acetylsalicylic acid (ASA; aspirin). Regular and frequent use (more than two to three times weekly) of these and other short-acting sedatives and anxiolytics as well as opioids should be avoided because of the potential for developing transform (rebound) headache, medication dependency or even addiction.

Occipital neuralgia. Pressure over occipital nerves or nerve injury due to trauma or surgery may activate headache symptoms. Nerve block may eliminate headache symptoms temporarily or for extended periods. Such blocks do not accurately predict the outcome of trial suboccipital nerve stimulation (see above).

Myofascial headache. Treatment includes awareness and avoidance of triggers, such as posture and stress. Analgesics are used with usual cautions. Trigger point injections may give short-term benefit, and physical therapy may be helpful.

Key points – headaches

- In patients without history of chronic headaches, determine whether an acute new headache is a serious, potentially life-threatening condition
- In chronic headache:
  - use a headache diary to differentiate headache type and establish pattern of triggers to enable self-management strategies
  - institute preventive measures such as trigger avoidance, stress control and medication
  - institute abortive regimen appropriate for headache type
    - migraine: NSAIDs, stress control, triptans
    - tension/myofascial: non-steroidal anti-inflammatory drugs, stress control, icing, stretching
  - avoid regular frequent analgesic use to reduce incidence of transform (rebound) headache physical dependency

Key references

Anon. The International Classification of Headache Disorders, 2nd edn. *Cephalalgia* 2004;24(suppl 1):9–160.

Ashina S, Lyngberg A, Jensen R. Headache characteristics and chronification of migraine and tension-type headache: A population-based study. *Cephalalgia* 2010;30:943–52.

Bigal ME, Ashina S, Burstein R et al. Prevalence and characteristics of allodynia in headache sufferers: a population study. *Neurology* 2008;70:1525–33.

Boardman HF, Thomas E, Millson DS, Croft PR. The natural history of headache: predictors of onset and recovery. *Cephalalgia* 2006;26:1080–8.

Francis GJ, Becker WJ, Pringsheim TM. Acute and preventive pharmacologic treatment of cluster headache. *Neurology* 2010;75:463–73.

Linde M. Migraine: a review and future directions for treatment. *Acta Neurol Scand* 2006;114:71–83.

Lipton RB, Silberstein SD, Saper JR et al. Why headache treatment fails. *Neurology* 2003;60:1064–70.

Loder E, Rizzoli P. Tension-type headache. *BMJ* 2008;336:88–92.

Maizels M, Burchette R. Rapid and sensitive paradigm for screening patients with headache in primary care settings. *Headache* 2003;43:441–50.

Merskey H, Bogduk N, eds. *Classification of Chronic Pain. Descriptions of Chronic Pain Syndromes and Definitions of Pain Terms*, 2nd edn. Seattle: IASP Press, 1994:77–94.

Ramadan NM, Silberstein SD, Freitag FG et al. *Evidence-Based Guidelines for Migraine Headache in the Primary Care Setting: Pharmacological Management for Prevention of Migraine*. American Academy of Neurology. http://pennfm.pbworks.com/f/ Migraine+Guidelines+-+Prevention. pdf, last accessed 5 Nov 2010.

Robbins MS, Grosberg BM, Napchan U et al. Clinical and prognostic subforms of new daily-persistent headache. *Neurology* 2010;74:1358–64.

12 The multidisciplinary approach and developments in pain management

The International Association for the Study of Pain (IASP), the American Academy of Pain Medicine, the Faculty of Pain Medicine of the Australian and New Zealand College of Anaesthetists and the American College of Rheumatology, among many other professional organizations, have long advocated the multidisciplinary approach as the preferred method of restoring health-related quality of life and functionality to patients with chronic pain, as it is a multidimensional condition.

The multidisciplinary team

The multidisciplinary (now often termed 'interdisciplinary', which implies an integration of treatments) approach to the treatment of chronic pain consists of assessing and treating the physical, psychosocial, medical, vocational and social aspects of chronic pain. The specific disciplines of healthcare providers required to offer multidisciplinary care are a function of the variety of patients seen and the available resources. The team may include physicians, nurses, psychologists, physical therapists, occupational therapists, vocational counselors, social workers, pharmacists and any other healthcare professional who can contribute to diagnosis and/or treatment.

Treatment is not 'one size fits all'. Ideally, treatment should selectively integrate different modalities following a goal-oriented management plan that is derived from a prioritized problem list based on a biopsychosocial formulation of the predisposing, precipitating and perpetuating factors of the presenting condition. It is crucial that the members of the treatment team communicate with each other on a regular basis, both about specific patients and about overall program development so that treatment is selectively targeted to achieve specific goals. Shared electronic medical records facilitate this process.

Research evidence to support the effectiveness of this approach to chronic pain treatment is just emerging. Meta-analyses of case-controlled cohort studies of the effectiveness of interdisciplinary care suggest that, in the case of disability from low back pain, such care increases rates of return to work and staying at work as compared with controls. However, researchers consistently stress the need to improve the number and the quality of the trials to evaluate the effectiveness of chronic pain treatment programs, particularly the selective integration of two or more treatments together. For example, much like in treating major depression, a combination of medication and cognitive therapy is superior to either therapy alone, and combining cognitive behavioral therapy and/or physical therapy with medication and/or injections should be superior to any one treatment; indeed, most 'clinical experts' recommend this approach.

Varied response for different syndromes. Systematic reviews of the literature suggest that the benefits of multidisciplinary therapy are not uniform across all chronic pain syndromes. For example, for patients with chronic low back pain, behavioral treatment such as positive reinforcement of healthy behaviors, modification of patients' understanding of their pain and disability, and biofeedback, all decrease pain intensity and improve functional status. Yet, in patients with chronic neck or shoulder pain or fibromyalgia, a similar approach lacks effectiveness.

The magnitude of the effect of a multidisciplinary approach ranges from slight to moderate. The benefits are less clear when a multidisciplinary approach supplements other standard treatment. For example, behavioral treatment for chronic low back pain has a moderate effect on pain intensity, functional status and behavioral outcomes compared with being on a waiting list or simply receiving no treatment. However, when added to a usual pharmacotherapy program for chronic low back pain the positive effect is not observed.

The intensity of the multidisciplinary program also seems relevant. For example, systematic reviews of trials that evaluate multidisciplinary therapy for chronic low back pain suggest that although intensive multidisciplinary biopsychosocial rehabilitation with a functional restoration approach reduces pain and improves

155

function, less intensive interventions do not produce improvement in any clinically relevant outcome.

Recent clinical trials of an interdisciplinary case management approach suggests that a stepped model of care, which establishes consultative/collaborative care for treatment resistance or complex cases, is cost-effective for low back pain in a primary care setting.

Further research. Because of the shortcomings in the methods used in published trials, the cost of multidisciplinary therapy and the increasing need to prove that the cost of proposed treatments is offset by the value they add, there is an obvious need for more research to demonstrate the benefits of this approach for the treatment of chronic pain.

Key points – the multidisciplinary approach

- As chronic pain is a multidimensional interdisciplinary biopsychosocial condition, expert consensus and some research recommends the multidisciplinary approach as the method of choice to restore quality of life and functionality.
- The specific disciplines of healthcare providers required to offer a multidisciplinary approach depend on the variety of patients seen and the available resources.
- Research evidence to support the effectiveness of the multidisciplinary or interdisciplinary approach to chronic pain treatment is not yet conclusive; there is an obvious need for more research to prove its cost-effectiveness.

Developments in pain management

Novel analgesics. The increased understanding of nociceptive transmission and pain pathophysiology, the recognition of heterogeneity among C fibers extending to their production of different molecular transducers, and the discovery of new receptors such as those for vanilloids or growth factors and identification of new receptor subtypes have already resulted in preclinical and early clinical testing of novel analgesics. These agents will more specifically target receptor subtypes or ion channels, and promise to be more effective and better tolerated than present therapies. Other novel molecules are designed to interact with multiple receptors simultaneously.

Advances in delivery. Setbacks that have followed the introduction of novel agents such as cyclooxygenase (COX)-2 inhibitors have been offset by the development of innovative methods to improve formulations of established compounds.

Iontophoretic or inhalational technology now permits the delivery of lipophilic opioids into the systemic circulation through the skin or lungs. Likewise, intranasal delivery of novel agents (or established agents coadministered with novel excipients) permits more rapid control of breakthrough pain than oral or transbuccal drug delivery.

Advances in imaging technology have taken us beyond a static detailed image of the central nervous system: we can now see the brain at work. Functional MRI allows real-time clinical observation of the brain's pain excitatory and inhibitory circuitry, which in turn helps us to understand how nociceptive input is processed and translated into pain and suffering. Functional imaging has advanced our knowledge of placebo and analgesic responses, and has even been applied as a novel form of biofeedback to allow patients to control their otherwise refractory chronic pain.

Magnetic resonance spectroscopy appears poised to achieve the Holy Grail of pain assessment: sensitive specific diagnosis of the presence of chronic pain using a quick simple laboratory test.

Pharmacogenetics. No doubt we will be using pharmacogenetics to prescribe analgesics in the future. Each medication will be tailored to the needs and characteristics of the individual, so that each patient will get the most benefit with the fewest side effects. Moreover, pharmacogenetics is already helping us to understand the biological basis for individual variability in response to established agents such as opioids.

Future hope. Individuals with chronic pain can look to the future with hope. Medical science has progressed from marginalizing chronic pain as merely a symptom of disease, and belittling those who seek help, to developing a better understanding of its causes and effects. Policy makers, including the World Health Organization, have come to realize the devastating effect that chronic pain has on individuals and their families, on society as a whole, and on the economy in terms of lost output and productivity.

Governments are accepting the importance of developing specialized strategies for the prevention, treatment and management of chronic pain as a fundamental human right, and are passing laws and regulations that encourage, and even mandate, improved systems of care for pain. In addition, health services around the world are responding to calls to improve the management of painful long-term conditions; to develop preventive and cost-effective solutions; to respond to patient choice and voice; and to create healthier workplaces (see www.painsummit.org.au). In 2010 an International Pain Summit was held for the first time at the IASP World Congress on Pain.

These advances should help individuals with chronic pain to overcome some of the problems they face in everyday life so that they can enjoy more opportunities, greater independence and an improved quality of life.

Key points – developments in pain management

- Increased understanding of chronic pain pathophysiology is leading to new pharmacological targets for treatment.
- New drugs will be more specific and promise to be more effective and to have fewer side effects.
- New methods of drug delivery are rapidly evolving.
- New imaging (especially of the brain) is providing new knowledge of central nervous system neuroplasticity changes.
- Pharmacogenetics holds out the possibility of specially tailored pharmacotherapy.

Key references

Multidisciplinary approach

Ang DC, Bair MJ, Damush TM et al. Predictors of pain outcomes in patients with chronic musculoskeletal pain co-morbid with depression: results from a randomized controlled trial. *Pain Med* 2010;11:482–91.

Deyo RA. *Back Pain Patient Outcomes Assessment Team (BOAT)*. Agency for Healthcare Research and Quality. www.ahcpr.gov/clinic/medtep/backpain.htm, last accessed 4 Nov 2010.

Dobscha SK, Corson K, Leibowitz RQ et al. Rationale, design, and baseline findings from a randomized trial of collaborative care for chronic musculoskeletal pain in primary care. *Pain Med* 2008;9:1050–64.

Gallagher RM. Biopsychosocial pain medicine and mind-brain-body science. *Phys Med Rehabil Clin N Am* 2004;15:855–82.

Gallagher RM. Treatment planning in pain medicine. Integrating medical, physical, and behavioral therapies. *Med Clin North Am* 1999;83:823–49.

Guzman J, Esmail R, Karjalainen K et al. Multidisciplinary biopsychosocial rehabilitation for chronic low back pain. *Cochrane Database Syst Rev* 2002, issue 1. CD000963. www.thecochranelibrary.com

Karjalainen K, Malmivaara A, van Tulder M et al. Biopsychosocial rehabilitation for upper limb repetitive strain injuries in working age adults. *Cochrane Database Syst Rev* 2000, issue 3. CD002269. www.thecochranelibrary.com

Karjalainen K, Malmivaara A, van Tulder M et al. Multidisciplinary rehabilitation for fibromyalgia and musculoskeletal pain in working age adults. *Cochrane Database Syst Rev* 2000, issue 2. CD001984. www.thecochranelibrary.com

Karjalainen K, Malmivaara A, van Tulder M et al. Multidisciplinary biopsychosocial rehabilitation for neck and shoulder pain among working age adults. *Cochrane Database Syst Rev* 2003, issue 2. CD002194. www.thecochranelibrary.com

Karjalainen K, Malmivaara A, van Tulder M et al. Multidisciplinary biopsychosocial rehabilitation for subacute low back pain among working age adults. *Cochrane Database Syst Rev* 2003, issue 2. CD002193. www.thecochranelibrary.com

Kroenke K, Bair MJ, Damush TM et al. Optimized antidepressant therapy and pain self-management in primary care patients with depression and musculoskeletal pain: a randomized controlled trial. *JAMA* 2009;301:2099–110.

National Pain Strategy. National Pain Summit of Australia. www.painsummit.org.au

Ostelo RW, van Tulder MW, Vlaeyen JW et al. Behavioural treatment for chronic low-back pain. *Cochrane Database Syst Rev* 2005, issue 1. CD002014. www.thecochranelibrary.com.

Developments in pain management

Bonney IM, Foran SE, Marchand JE et al. Spinal antinociceptive effects of AA501, a novel chimeric peptide with opioid receptor agonist and tachykinin receptor antagonist moieties. *Eur J Pharmacol* 2004;488:91–9.

Cousins MJ, Brennan F, Carr DB. Pain relief: a universal human right. *Pain* 2004;112:1–4.

Dubois MY, Gallagher RM, Lippe PM. Pain medicine position paper. *Pain Med* 2009;10:972–1000.

Gordon DB, Dahl JL, Miaskowski C et al. American pain society recommendations for improving the quality of acute and cancer pain management: American Pain Society Quality of Care Task Force. *Arch Intern Med* 2005;165:1574–80.

Kim H, Dionne RA. Genetics, pain, and analgesia. *Pain: Clinical Updates* 2005, vol XIII. www.iasp-pain.org/ AM/AMTemplate.cfm?Section= Home&TEMPLATE=/CM/ ContentDisplay.cfm& CONTENTID=7637, last accessed 4 Nov 2010.

Siddall PJ, Cousins MJ. Persistent pain as a disease entity: implications for clinical management. *Anesth Analg* 2004;99:510–20.

Siddall PJ, Stanwell P, Woodhouse A et al. Magnetic resonance spectroscopy detects biochemical changes in the brain associated with chronic low back pain: a preliminary report. *Anesth Analg* 2006;102:1164–8.

Stamer UM, Stuber F. Pharmacogenetics of anesthetic and analgesic agents: CYP2D6 genetic variations. *Anesthesiology* 2005;103:1099; author reply 101.

Veterans Health Administration. Pain management. *VHA Directive 2009-053*, 2009. www.va.gov/ PAINMANAGEMENT/docs/ VHA09PainDirective.pdf, last accessed 4 Nov 2010.

Villanueva L, Dickenson A, Ollat H, eds. *The Pain System in Normal and Pathological States: A Primer for Clinicians*. Seattle: IASP Press, 2004.

Useful resources

Cousins MJ, Carr DB, Horlocker T, Bridenbaugh PO, eds. *Neural Blockade in Clinical Anesthesia & Pain Medicine*, 4th edn. Philadelphia: Wolters Kluwer/ Lippincott, Williams & Wilkins, 2009.

Specifically, the following chapters:

Binder A, Baron R. Complex regional pain syndrome including applications of neural blockade, pp 1154–68.

Burton AW, Phan PC, Cousins MJ. Treatment of cancer pain, pp 1111–53.

Carr DB, Cousins MJ. Spinal route of analgesia, pp 886–947.

Niv D, Gofeld M. Percutaneous neural destructive techniques, pp 991–1035.

Prager JP, Stanton-Hicks M. Neurostimulation, pp 948–90.

Siddall PJ, Cousins MJ. Introduction to pain mechanisms: implications for neural blockade, pp 661–92.

Vije C, Ashburn M A. Assessment and diagnosis of chronic pain conditions, pp 801–10.

Useful addresses

UK
The British Pain Society
Tel: +44 (0)20 7269 7840
info@britishpainsociety.org
www.britishpainsociety.org

Chronic Pain Policy Coalition
Tel: +44 (0)20 7202 8580
info@paincoalition.org.uk
www.paincoalition.org.uk

Pain Concern
Tel: +44 (0)1620 822572
(Mon–Fri 9 AM–5 PM)
info@painconcern.org.uk
www.painconcern.org.uk

The Pain Relief Foundation
Tel: +44 (0)151 529 5820
secretary@painrelieffoundation.org.uk
www.painrelieffoundation.org.uk

USA
Agency for Healthcare Research and Quality
Tel: +1 301 427 1104
www.ahrq.gov

Alliance of State Pain Initiatives
Tel: +1 608 265 4013
aspi@mailplus.wisc.edu
www.aspi.wisc.edu

American Academy of Neurology
Tel: +1 651 695 2717
Toll-free: 800 879 1960
www.aan.com

American Academy of
Orofacial Pain
Tel: +1 856 423 3629
aaopco@talley.com
www.aaop.org

American Academy of Pain
Medicine
Tel: +1 847 375 4731
info@painmed.org
www.painmed.org

American Chronic Pain
Association
Toll-free: 800 533 3231
ACPA@pacbell.net
www.theacpa.org

American Pain Foundation
Toll-free: 1 888 615 7246
info@painfoundation.org
www.painfoundation.org

American Pain Society
Tel: +1 847 375 4715
info@ampainsoc.org
www.ampainsoc.org

Partners Against Pain
Toll-free: 888 726 7535
medical_services@pharma.com
www.partnersagainstpain.com

Trigeminal Neuralgia Association
Toll-free: +1 800 923 3608
Tel: +1 352 331 7009
www.fpa-support.org

International
Australian Pain Society
Tel: +61 (0)2 9954 4400
www.apsoc.org.au

Canadian Pain Society
Tel: +1 905 404 9545
www.canadianpainsociety.ca

European Federation of IASP
Chapters
Tel: +32 2 251 55 10
secretary@efic.org
www.efic.org

Faculty of Pain Medicine of the
Australian and New Zealand
College of Anaesthetists
Tel: +61 (0)3 8517 5337
painmed@anzca.edu.au
www.anzca.edu.au/fpm

International Association for the
Study of Pain
Tel: +1 206 283 0311
iaspdesk@iasp-pain.org
www.iasp-pain.org

International MYOPAIN Society
(Myofascial pain and
Fibromyalgia Syndrome)
Tel: +1 210 401 7224
www.myopain.org

International Pelvic Pain Society
Tel: +1 847 517 8712
info@pelvicpain.org
www.pelvicpain.org

Pain South Africa
Tel/Fax: +27 (0)43 642 1928
info@painsa.co.za
www.pain-management.co.za

Trigeminal Neuralgia Association
of Canada
Tel: +1 403 327 7668
president@tnac.org
www.tnac.org

Other useful resources
Australian National Health and
Medical Research Council
*Acute Pain Management: Scientific
Evidence* 3rd edn, 2010. Available
from www.nhmrc.gov.au/
publications/synopses/cp104syn.
htm

Bandolier
www.medicine.ox.ac.uk/bandolier

National Institute for Health
and Clinical Excellence
(England & Wales)
www.nice.org.uk
*Neuropathic Pain. The
pharmacological management of
neuropathic pain in adults in
non-specialist settings*. Full
Guidelines CG96. NICE, 2010.
Available from http://guidance.nice.
org.uk/CG96/Guidance/pdf/English

Index

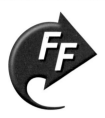

Fast Facts – the ultimate medical handbook series covers 72 topics, including:

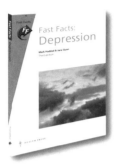

Fast Facts:
Depression

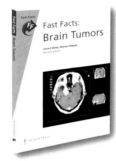

Fast Facts:
Brain Tumors

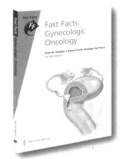

Fast Facts:
Gynecologic Oncology

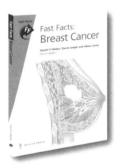

Fast Facts:
Breast Cancer

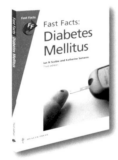

Fast Facts:
Diabetes Mellitus

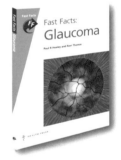

Fast Facts:
Glaucoma

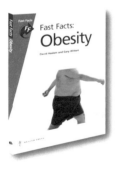

Fast Facts:
Obesity

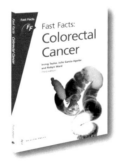

Fast Facts:
Colorectal Cancer

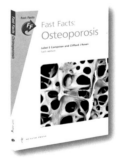

Fast Facts:
Osteoporosis

www.fastfacts.com